A Late Diagnosis
of Autism

How to Help Your Newly Diagnosed
Autie Survive the Challenges of Ageing,
Illness and Everyday Life

Shonagh Mackie

Published by New Generation Publishing in 2024

Copyright © Shonagh Mackie 2024

First Edition

The author asserts the moral right under the Copyright, Designs and Patents Act 1988 to be identified as the author of this work.

All Rights reserved. No part of this publication may be reproduced, stored in a retrieval system or transmitted, in any form or by any means without the prior consent of the author, nor be otherwise circulated in any form of binding or cover other than that which it is published and without a similar condition being imposed on the subsequent purchaser.

shonaghmackie@outlook.com
https://linkedin.com/company/shonagh-mackie

ISBN: 978-1-83563-425-7

www.newgeneration-publishing.com
New Generation Publishing

Praise for A Late Diagnosis of Autism (before publication)

"I think it's a great book. Very impressive. You cover a lot of ground and it's written in an accessible but not over-simplistic way. I would be happy to buy a copy and recommend it to the folk we see at Number 6."

Tim Hather, Number 6 One-Stop Shop, a service provided by Autism Initiatives UK

"This book is very much needed and so overdue… it will be so enlightening for many of my clients. It helps me understand more and more about autism and with Mack being so open and honest (and funny!), during counselling sessions, it has given me further insight into just how many areas of life can be impacted by autism and also just how much more there is for us to still learn."

Suneeta Gogna, Oceanic Counselling

"Wow – this has really moved on a notch – especially the later sections. It's so much more revealing about the struggles that I feel it will really help the neurotypical family members to survive too! A book I read many years ago on living with a ND partner said either to learn to accommodate or get a divorce – there was no mid-way. What I find particularly powerful is that you now encompass much more of the 'stuff' no-one is talking about for the 60-ish year olds who have never been accommodated."

Sabrina, wife of a recently diagnosed Autie and mother of another (both AuDHD)

"I love the writing style. It really hooks you in and makes you want to keep reading. As a foster carer to many children of all ages, sometimes it's hard to work out what is usual teenage grumpy, difficult, to be expected behaviour, and what could genuinely be them struggling with situations. Reading this book I had several lightbulb moments which gave me pause to think about how I could have better handled situations. Only wish I had read this years ago."

Marina, foster mum of a now-adult autistic son

"Wish I'd had something like this to read when my friend/colleague first told me she was autistic several years ago. Instead, I waded my way through a few dry text books and still came away with misconceptions. Although she's different from Mack in some ways, in other ways this explains her perfectly which is so helpful! I also now understand why her symptoms have been getting worse as we've gotten older – increased anxiety and exhaustion in particular. However, I now not only have some more ideas of how I can be more accommodating, I've discovered lots of things I should stop doing that have probably been making her life more difficult! Thank you for sharing."

Lesley, friend and colleague of an Autie diagnosed several years ago

Dedication

To Stuart and Halle, whose very existence makes each day in their father's life better than the last. May you always find meaning and happiness in your own lives.

Disclaimers

The names of individuals mentioned in this journal have been changed to protect their privacy.

At the time of writing, there's little information available about autism in adults – or age-related aspects of autism such as late-in-life burnout or coping with illness and the ageing process. However, new research is being done every day, and we hope that, say, a decade from now our understanding of autism in adults will be infinitely better than it is now. Meantime, while this journal has been reviewed by fellow travellers and professionals working in the fields of autism and psychology, its findings are based on information available to us during our investigations, and the experiences and opinions expressed are ours alone unless clearly stated otherwise.

And finally, while we've attempted to recall events as accurately as our fading memories allow, in the words of Her Late Majesty Queen Elizabeth, "recollections may vary".

Contents

Foreword 1
Sensory issues 6
   Sensory sensitivity 6
   Interoception 14
   Medication sensitivity 22
Communication issues 27
   Social communication difficulties 27
   Listening 35
   Telepathy 43
Interaction and anxiety 49
   General anxiety 49
   Social anxiety 57
   Meltdowns 64
   Self-worth 70
   Depression 78
   Trauma 86
   Gastro issues 89
   Medical anxiety 94
   Catastrophising 101
   Stimming 106
   Repetitive behaviour 108
   Rules 114
Other differences 120
   Memory 120

- Learning and working things out 127
- Persevering and perseverating 135
- Uncertainty 141
- Empathy 149
- Integrity 156
- Enthusiasms and special interests 160
- Gifts 167
- Clumsiness 173
- Punctuality 180
- Impulsiveness 185
- Compulsiveness 191

Coping with illness 196
- Diagnosis 196
- Treatment 206
- Recovery 221

Back to life 234
- The crash and burn 234
- Beyond the wall 240
- Strategies for Mack 244
- Strategies for me 252
- Explaining it to others 259
- The future 261

Epilogue 263

Acknowledgements 286

Foreword

My husband Mack was diagnosed as autistic at the age of 63. Yes, *63*! I still can't imagine how he managed to mask his struggles for that length of time, but eventually he reached the stage where he was no longer able to hide the very real toll it was taking on his health. Psychologically, it was as though he'd hit a stone wall, at speed. And I had no idea what was happening to him or how to help.

I think it was his daughter Halle who first mentioned the word 'autism', at least *half*-joking. Out of curiosity, she chivvied us all into completing the autism-spectrum quotient test (AQ50) online and we laughed about his having 'aced' it, believing he must have cheated. And then we forgot about it. Many months later, Mack was blethering to local stonemason Iain who, out of nowhere, said to him, "You're autistic too, aren't you" – a statement not a question. That really gave us pause for thought.

Mack had been struggling with both his physical and mental health for a while, so during a consultation at his GP practice he was asked by the psychiatric nurse to complete a ream of questionnaires – for depression and trauma as well as autism – and was referred for an autism diagnosis. And that's when we began our fascinating journey to understanding his different neurology – and understanding *him*.

Following the diagnosis Mack was offered invaluable support by Number 6, a Scottish charity providing a 'one-stop shop' service for autistic adults. By taking part in a course of weekly online sessions with other recently diagnosed Auties, he learned way more about autism and how to manage the implications than we'd gleaned from weeks of googling and reading. I know Mack found the sessions invaluable, but even though he'd tell me after each one about the things he'd learned, I still struggled to understand how best to support his efforts to return to living what I'd call 'a full life' after the wall.

Most of the resources I'd found seemed to be for or about people across the spectrum or were written for parents of autistic children. And although they were fascinating and thought-provoking, I struggled to find anything that spoke to *me* as a family member about how to support my own newly unveiled but undeniably mature Autie.

What I needed, over and above an explanation of autism, was some kind of instruction manual on handling vintage Auties. Particularly the type who are so accomplished that they could successfully bluff their way through six decades of life with no one suspecting anything was off-kilter.

And that's why we decided to delve deep into Mack's life and uncover all the different ways autism affects him, journaling the conclusions of our discoveries. I hope this will help me, firstly, to think through all we've been learning so that I can better support Mack and, secondly, to properly explain it to other family members and friends – rather than leave them thinking he's bizarrely morphed into an over-anxious recluse. Perhaps it could help the families and friends of other newly diagnosed Auties too, we'll see. I'm a great starter, but not so much of a finisher!

So, from a starting point of nigh on complete ignorance, the first thing I learned is that Auties' brains are *wired* differently to other people's. And that while not all Auties are the same, they usually all experience some differences in sensory sensitivities, social communication and social interaction. The late diagnosis group sessions Mack took part in discussed and explained all those differences, most of which affect Mack to a greater or lesser extent.

Together, he and I have sifted our way through all this information extensively to develop our understanding of the impact his autism has had – and continues to have – on his life, and to decide what we should do going forward to make life easier. For both of us.

Before I begin though: a health warning. The facilitator of Mack's sessions warned the group that they may want to take some time to get their heads round their own diagnoses before telling other people – to truly understand it themselves first. It's not necessarily that people are judgy, but that everyday folk just don't know that much about it and will make assumptions about you based on what little information or *mis*information they have. Or on stereotypes portrayed on TV or film – Rain Man, Mercury Rising, The Imitation Game for example. Until you've had time to understand it yourself, you're not going to be much good at explaining it to *them*.

It's true to say I knew very little about autism before Mack's diagnosis. To the best of my knowledge, I'd only ever met two Auties before, and I only recognise this in retrospect. One of those people was a colleague of mine, the other a colleague of Mack's. Two things stood out about them. The first, they were both very clever; the second, (unlike Mack) they had absolutely no social graces whatsoever!

And I had assumed that was pretty much all there was to it: Auties were smart and socially a bit dysfunctional. Quintessentially, gifted eccentrics or quirky geeks.

Other people however, rightly or wrongly believe all sorts of things about autism which have caused them concern and possibly resulted in them misunderstanding Mack completely. That's my fault; I was so relieved to have an explanation for his increasing agoraphobia that I'd told a few people before we'd worked it through and found a succinct way to explain it. And actually, does anyone really need to know at all? I guess that should be entirely the Autie's choice.

I'm not sure whether either of the Auties I mentioned had ever been diagnosed. Quite rightly, people just accepted them the way they were, foibles'n all.

>   <<My colleague – let's call him Donald – had been a frenemy for many years before he came to work for me. The team undoubtedly found him difficult, but they respected his knowledge and learned to put up with his abruptness.
>
>   It was tricky with clients though. Someone would call to explain a complex issue they were facing and ask whether their proposed solution was within the scope of the rules and regulations. Donald would patiently listen, say "No" and then simply put the phone down!
>
>   Affronted by his manner, many clients refused to deal with him. My response to them was along the lines of, "That's no problem. I'm sure Donald didn't mean to be rude or difficult; it's just that he's 'a little autistic'. I can give you a perfectly capable and genial account manager instead, or you can stick with one of the smartest and most knowledgeable compliance professionals in the country." That usually worked!>>
>
>   Mack

Oh, the irony! Sadly, Donald is no longer with us, but I'm sure he'll be having a good chuckle from the hereafter –

Mack being diagnosed as autistic would definitely have appealed to his very dry sense of humour.

By the time we've completed this foray into understanding autism, we hope to be able to explain its effect on Mack clearly and simply, focusing on the advantages at least as much as on the drawbacks. And to have developed a much better strategy for living life as we enter retirement.

Sensory issues

Sensory sensitivity

10 December

I was astounded to discover that sensory sensitivity is an aspect of autism – and a huge one too. I had no idea, although I should have had because there have been plenty of clues along the way.

For instance, we'd be in a supermarket or hardware store and Mack would inexplicably abandon the trolley and shoot towards the exit while shielding his eyes. He won't stay in a restaurant or bar if it's busy or echoey – we have to about-turn quick smart. And he's hyperaware of all sorts of things – "What was that sound?", "Can you smell something funny?", "Did you feel that?"

My mother jokes about him being neurotic sometimes, but usually it turns out that there *is* actually something to hear (a scurrying mouse), smell (damp or a dead rat) or feel (a dodgy electric blanket) that we ought perhaps to be worried about after all. As a sniffer, he could put our cocker spaniel grandpuppy Haggis to shame.

The trouble seems to be when there's just way too much to sense or take in. Let's say we're meeting friends for lunch. I walk into the restaurant, scan the room looking for them and make my way over to their table. I haven't really clocked anything else. But Mack has already taken in the layout, the aromas, the number of diners, the noise level, where the gents is, the colour of the napkins, the nearest escape route…

If there's too much activity, too many people or too much noise, his head explodes and he has to leave.

And to the bewildered left behind, I say, "Oh…, he just had to step out to take an urgent business call…" (Not that this excuse will wash for much longer with retirement looming!)

😮 **Autistic people can experience hypersensitivity, which can result in sensory overload – hence the rushing out of shops and restaurants. This constantly being hyperaware is incredibly exhausting.**

> <<It happens a lot, abandoning trolleys or baskets – sometimes you just *have* to get out.
>
> I was in a DIY store a few years ago and I had about three trolley loads of kitchen units and related bits and pieces. It was busy, it was echoey, the queue was taking ages and the lighting in the store was horrendous. I could feel my eyes spacing out and that made me start to panic, thinking I was going to faint – I just had to make a break for it! I can still hear them shouting after me – boy, were they cross!>>
>
> Mack

It seems this isn't unusual. Mack tells me that all the others taking part in his online group sessions had exactly the same problem and similar stories to tell about both shopping and eating out. Thankfully, I don't remember Mack ever doing a runner in the middle of a meal. He's more likely to opt out at the threshold – or at worst once we've sat down but before we've ordered. Though now that I think about it, he's very keen to leave as soon as he's taken his last mouthful.

He's always been choosy about where to sit in a restaurant. He hates to be in the middle of the fray with noise and hustle'n bustle all around, and if changing tables or swapping seats isn't an option, it's more than likely we won't be staying. For Mack, that would be an experience to be endured rather than enjoyed. And I guess that's why you're way more likely to find us munching a sandwich in the car than sitting in a café for lunch.

As for shopping, DIY stores tend to be far less busy than supermarkets, so his trips there are less likely to result in a ditch and dash. Although it still happens. It's generally just the lighting and the echoey noises that cause him problems there.

While he finds fluorescent lights – or energy saving lights with a green hue or flicker – are best avoided, if lighting does trigger a reaction, Mack reaches straight for the sunglasses and paracetamol.

One of the tips Mack was given by Number 6 was to try wearing earplugs when out and about. He was sceptical at first, but popped in his AirPods for a trip to the supermarket one day and was astonished at the difference it made. So we've invested in proper earplugs!

> <<The difference really was incredible. They cut out so much of the extraneous noise that I hadn't even appreciated was getting to me.
>
> I'd attributed most of the stress I felt in stores to the people, and to potentially having to wait in a queue. And that definitely does stress me out. But with the sounds of the fridges and freezers, air-conditioning, beeping and general hubbub subdued, the experience was remarkably different.
>
> Somehow I found it much easier to navigate – the earplugs didn't seem to affect my awareness of what was happening in the

immediate vicinity, and I could still hear but without feeling that I was being assaulted by other people's conversations.

It wasn't busy – there were only about three people in the veg isle – and I was literally in and out for a few items, but I was quite happy to take my time and even stopped for a chat with the beggar at the door on the way out.>>

Mack

Another invaluable tip Mack was given was to rest his senses frequently to ease the sensory burden. Think super-catnap. Or if, for example, he's having a meal out or a drink with friends, to take a couple of loo breaks and give himself a few minutes of peace and quiet in a solitary cubicle. A little odd maybe, but if it works for others it sounds well worth trying!

11 December

☹ **That there was such a thing as sensory sensitivity blew my mind. But if we can take account of Mack's sensitivities, it could really open up the world for him again.**

Takeaways for Mack
- Avoid places with flickering lights and keep a pair of sunglasses in the car for use just in case.
- Stash earplugs in useful places – in the car, in jacket pockets – so they're handy whenever he needs them for muffling background noise.
- Make up a sensory emergency kit containing everything that helps stave off overload – earplugs, sunglasses or eye mask, paracetamol, calm-me-down meds, etc.

- Find less noisy, crowded venues whenever possible in favour of more sensory friendly places.
- Take super-catnaps or breaks whenever he starts to flag.

Takeaways for me
- Believe him when he says he smells or hears something that worries him, because it turns out he's not paranoid after all.
- Cut him some slack when it comes to the types of environment that are likely to give him overload – this should be much easier now that we understand what's causing the problem.
- Choose quiet venues with non-flickering or subdued lighting, good sound absorption and clear escape routes.
- In a pub, café or restaurant, give him a seat in a corner or with his back to a wall if possible so that his senses are only being assaulted from one direction.
- In a train, plane, theatre or cinema, book an aisle seat.

12 December

I mentioned that constantly being hyperaware is incredibly exhausting. It took me a while to get my head round that, but it explains why Mack is so tired by the time he gets home from pretty much any excursion. The Autie brain simply can't filter things out the way the neurotypical brain can.

I tend to focus on where I'm going and what I'm going there for, to the exclusion of all the extraneous stuff. So I would only notice lighting if, for example, it failed. My eyes search out the people I'm looking for or the items I want to buy without taking in the faces of other people or the features of other items. While I'd hear an 'excuse me', I don't notice peripheral sounds such as babbling voices, whining children, wailing car alarms, pinging mobiles, whirring air-conditioning, beeping scanners or payment machines, clinking cans or cutlery…

I could bump into someone, say sorry and walk on by without having registered a single thing about them. While I might be able to tell you whether it had been a hulking great man or a small child, I'd struggle to be any more explicit. I'd make a hopeless witness! Mack, on the other hand, would probably be able to describe the person's appearance and distinguishing features as well as details of what they were wearing or carrying, and would no doubt be able to pick them out in a line-up.

It's not just sight and sound that are affected by this sensory sensitivity; many Auties have issues with touch and smell too.

I have some silicone freezer bags for storing food, the sight of which makes Mack shudder or squirm because he can't stand the feel of them. And there are lots of foods he won't eat for a similar reason – sweet potato is way too 'slimy', just-ripened bananas too 'dry', kiwi fruit too 'crawly' – and the waft of a lovely tikka masala or pesto dish puts him right off whatever he's eating. Mind you, I feel the same about the texture of liver or kidney and the smell of kedgeree – maybe I should check my own AQ score again…

I used to wear perfume occasionally, and I'm only now realising that I stopped doing that probably not long after Mack appeared in my life. I don't think it's something he ever mentioned or complained about; I just became aware that he never wore smellies of any kind himself and that he seemed to prefer unscented everything. I presumed this was to do with skin sensitivity, but perhaps it was more to do with olfactory sensitivity.

Thankfully, his smell and texture issues aren't life-limiting in any way!

Oh, and then there's balance – I'd forgotten about that, but I'm pretty sure this is something that would come under sensory sensitivity too. And it's something that seems to have become worse with age – particularly when it comes to ladders.

We'd not long taken possession of our rural weekend bolthole when Mack started complaining about feeling a bit woozy from time to time. He found the second bedroom (which we were planning to use as a study) particularly bad. Until he had a lightbulb moment and said, "Is it just me, or is this floor off?" Off? What on earth was he talking about?

So he put a pencil down on the floor and, right enough, it rolled away. And that's when the spirit level came out... Several months later and pretty much every room in the house had been tackled – a new beam here, an extra joist there, and flooring levelled everywhere. As you can imagine, it cost a fortune. But at least he's flat and happy now, and he's made a great pal of the joiner. Yes, we can recommend a terrific joiner should you ever need one.

While there's a huge downside to this sensory sensitivity – i.e. the constant risk of overload and exhaustion – there's a flipside too. It's also a superpower.

It's night-time, we're both still awake, he'll say, "Did you hear that? What *was* that?" I listen, hear nothing, and then, "Oh! It's a tawny owl!" I'd never have heard it if he hadn't prompted me to listen out for it.

I'm cooking mince/bolognese sauce on the hob, I get distracted, wander off... 10 minutes later he'll say, "What's that smell?!" I sniff, sniff again and, "Oh, crap!" But it's usually just in time – virtually dry but not *quite* burnt yet.

He'll also spot the smallest things I'd otherwise miss – a cheeky wren looking to set up home inside our jerry-built pallet picnic table, an old friend in the crowd at the other side of a park (I could pass my mother in the street and not notice!) or a weevil in a sandwich he's just bought. In many ways, he's a very handy person to have around!

>> <<It's a pain when people won't believe you when you tell them something's wrong.

> A bunch of us were having a drink at a nearby pub-restaurant after work one summer evening, sitting outdoors under warmers (it is Scotland after all), and I could feel a tingling down my spine. I couldn't pinpoint what was wrong at first. And then I wondered if there was an odd smell over and above the usual aromas of beer and curry, so I said, "Can anyone else smell that?"

> They looked at me, sniffed, looked at each other, said "Nope" and carried on their conversation. But there was definitely something not right.

> "Are you sure you can't smell… gas, or something?" Again, they paused, sniffed and carried on. By now, I'm standing up and wandering around, sniffing as discreetly as one can. They tell me to sit down, which I reluctantly do. But only a few minutes later there was a bang immediately followed by a burning inferno! Of course, we all jumped and scattered like startled pigeons, but my first thought thereafter was along the lines of a rather childish "*Told* you so!">>

> Mack

Interoception

14 December

Mack will often become dehydrated and complain, "I just don't have a thirst reflex." I roll my eyes because that sounds plain daft to me. Plus, you drink intermittently through the day out of sheer habit if nothing else, don't you? He'll take his jumper off, put it back on, then take it off again and say, "Is it hot or is it cold in here?" – and his clammy hands are freezing. Sometimes, he'll be pale, wobbly and feeling faint – turns out he's had virtually nothing to eat since breakfast time, but he thinks he's coming down with something.

Between you and me, I've always rubber-eared the temperature thing and found the not eating and drinking enough a little exasperating. Shame on me. But to be fair, I had to look up 'interoception' as I'd never even heard of it before.

Interoception is about how you perceive sensations from inside your body. And it's a 'thing'. A real verifiable scientific thing as well as something Auties can have problems with.

The first hit I found when researching interoception was an article in The Guardian called *Interoception: the hidden sense that shapes wellbeing*[1]. I found it fascinating. It explained that interoception includes all the signals from your internal organs, including your cardiovascular system, your lungs, your gut, your bladder and your kidneys.

---

[1] The Guardian (2021), Interoception: the hidden sense that shapes wellbeing. Accessed December 2022 at:
https://www.theguardian.com/science/2021/aug/15/the-hidden-sense-shaping-your-wellbeing-interoception

Signals we (neurotypical people) generally all receive and interpret correctly without even realising.

Before reading up on interoception, I was only aware of the five senses I'd learned about in my school days – sight, sound, taste, touch and smell. But our investigations uncovered three further sensory systems – vestibular (to do with balance), proprioception (to do with movement) and interoception (to do with how you feel) – and shows that people can be hy*po* or hy*per*sensitive to any of the eight.

So gone are the days when the sixth sense alluded to ghosts. Which must have been a big disappointment to Bruce Willis and Haley Joel Osment.

Interoception doesn't just send messages from your organs to tell you about body matters – such as hunger, thirst, the need to go to the loo, pain and fatigue – it covers emotional states too. For example, anxiety, anger, irritability, fear, sadness, excitement or joy.

So if you have problems with interoception awareness, you could easily confuse some of these signals. I admit that occasionally I think I'm hungry, but because I know I can't be – I had a huge lunch – I know it must actually be thirst. It's a bit daunting to think that some people's confusion must be more significant than that. What would it be like not to be sure whether you were in pain or needed the loo? Whether it was irritability or excitement you were feeling? Or not being able to tell the difference between sadness and fatigue?

Thankfully, Mack doesn't have issues with all of these things – just thirst, temperature, hunger sometimes, tiredness and some emotions. It's the emotions that are still a bit of an unknown at this point. I know he often feels anxiety and sadness, but I don't know to what extent – if any – he's misreading those feelings. Bear with me on this one as I know it's a bit whacky – but what if the anxiety and sadness he feels is nothing of the sort? What if his body is actually telling him he's excited and hungry?

OK, maybe that's a step too far, but nothing wrong with keeping an open mind!

A little further delving threw up the term alexithymia. I have no idea how to even pronounce it, but that's what you call the difficulty some people have in identifying and articulating emotions. If you can't describe your feelings and put words to them, then you can't explain your emotional state. This is one of the reasons why counselling can be difficult for Auties.

Let's assume Mack *does* interpret his emotions correctly – we don't have any evidence to suggest otherwise after all – but that he's just not reading the signals soon enough. I guess that would work just the same way as the temperature problem. By the time he's sure that he's cold rather than hot, he's actually freezing. This might explain why he doesn't recognise tiredness, for example, until he's absolutely wiped out. Which, now that I think about it, is almost a daily occurrence.

It doesn't matter how often I say during the day, "Slow down", "Don't overdo it" or even "Stop, you've had enough", he just rubber-ears me. "Yeah, I'm fine, I'll just get this finished…" I always swore as a child that I've never become an I-told-you-so person, but for goodness' sake!

This is probably quite key to understanding Mack's emotional responses in certain situations. If you don't realise you're stressed, tired or angry until you're snapping, crying or breaking something, that emotion has gone beyond the point where you can control it easily. If you'd realised sooner, you could have walked away, taken a few deep breaths or a rest and been OK. This is a nut we really need to figure out how to crack.

15 December

Most of the information I could find on interoception and autism suggested a complex picture. I guess it goes back to no two Auties are the same but, in general, autistic people seem to read their body signals less well than neurotypical people but have more interoceptive sensitivity – which means a greater awareness or exaggerated perception of bodily sensations.

☺ **Studies show that autistic people tend not to read their body's signals well. Learning to read these signals better could be key to improving their sense of wellbeing.**

> <<I've always had problems remembering to drink, and sometimes with judging my temperature, but I didn't realise this was a 'thing', and in the past doctors had been very dismissive when I mentioned not being able to tell when I was thirsty.
>
> Now, this stuff makes sense. It explains why I have such a hard time pinpointing what's wrong when I'm not feeling well, why sometimes I forget to eat or drink – especially when I'm preoccupied – and why I can suddenly feel overcome with anxiety and tiredness out of nowhere.>>
>
> Mack

I can't even imagine not realising you're hungry, thirsty or cold – it's amazing to me. So the suggestion that you could do something to develop an awareness came as a relief.

And that's what led me to 'mindfulness' – a wellbeing approach I also knew nothing about. I fear that for many it may conjure up images of happy hippies, incense and dancing at the summer solstice, but when I googled it the first hit actually came from the NHS[2]. And you can't get a more solid recommendation than that.

According to them, mindfulness is about connecting with our bodies and the sensations they experience. It's about developing a greater awareness by paying close attention to the sights, sounds, smells, tastes, thoughts and feelings of the present moment.

Mindfulness meditation in particular sounds as though it would help develop interoception, as this involves sitting silently and concentrating on the sensations of breathing and parts of the body. Through mindfulness, you should be able to train yourself to recognise the body's signals better.

😲 **Wow. Just wow.**

My one concern about this is that Mack has tried hypnotherapy before, with zero success. Something to do with being unable to relax or relinquish control. So, pessimistically, I'm not holding my breath about him being able to master mindfulness.

---

[2] NHS (2022), Mindfulness. Accessed December 2022 at: **https://www.nhs.uk/mental-health/self-help/tips-and-support/mindfulness**

Takeaways for Mack
- Set reminders to drink throughout the day – and act on them. (Newsflash Mack, pouring a drink isn't the same as actually *drinking* it!)
- When a slump hits, eat something.
- Avoid slumps by eating more frequently. For example, elevenses, threeses and supper as well as breakfast, lunch and dinner. Routine helps.
- Try mindfulness exercises from time to time, concentrating on reading body signals. If he draws the curtains he may feel less of a numpty!

Takeaways for me
- If he's not eating and drinking whenever I am, nag him. Gently or otherwise.
- Encourage him to do exercises to improve his ability to read these body signals.

<<I guess I could try the meditation thing.

I find open water therapeutic and have often gone to sit at the seashore or riverside when I've felt particularly down. There's something soothing about the sound of lapping water or waves – it allows you to empty your mind, which would be a good place to start.>>

Mack

16 December

The article I mentioned also claimed that interoception lies behind our sense of intuition – when something feels 'right' or 'wrong' without an explanation.

I can't find much on this, but I know that Mack does a lot of things based on his 'feelings'. Usually, he'll try to find a reason for feelings before acting on them, but will just rely on gut instinct if he can't figure it out. That might mean battening down the hatches if he thinks there's a storm coming (we'd usually be able to check on that). Or he'll be convinced the car's not quite right and spend hours fiddling about underneath or under the bonnet trying to get to the bottom of it. The car could be in bits before he actually finds anything wrong! But maybe that's saved our lives at one point, who knows.

There was at least one occasion when he made me take my car to the garage and, right enough, they found something that had become dangerous. While I can no longer remember what it was (a broken spring?), I *do* remember he blew his horn about it for weeks! And there was another time when he kept going on about a vibration. I couldn't feel anything, but when humming along to the radio I did notice that I sounded remarkably like a dalek on helium!

He also gets déjà-vu. I think a lot of people experience that sometimes. You're walking down the street and a smell from the past hits you (granny's perfume, great-grandad's pipe-smoke, the creosote from the potting shed of your childhood) and suddenly you're back there. Mack tells me he experiences it often in conversations, when he knows exactly what someone's about to say. I expect there's a scientific explanation for all of it, and it may well be to do with hyperawareness, interoception and the simple fact that his wiring means he uses different parts of his brain differently.

>> <<My uncle died a few years ago, and of course I wanted to be at the funeral. However, I had a niggling anxiety about going, which felt like something over and above the thought of the five-hour car journey and an overnight stay. I just couldn't pin it down.

Shonagh assured me she'd look after Dad while I was away, and he assured me he'd be fine, and so I reluctantly set off along with my sister Eilidh the evening before.

Like a mother hen, I phoned several times to make sure everything was OK because that nagging feeling wouldn't go away. Right enough, as the evening went on Dad began to feel unwell. By 10pm Shonagh had called NHS 24, by midnight a doctor was there and by 8am Dad was carted into hospital by ambulance.

Needless to say, we never made it to my uncle's funeral – we hit the road straight back home the moment we woke up to the news.>>

Mack

Medication sensitivity

19 December

When I was a student, I wanted to give blood but there was a sign at the door that effectively said don't bother if you're under eight stone. I was about six and a half stone in those days. I've never noticed any medication dosage being altered to account for being a sparrow though – there's generally just a standard adult dose or a child dose. This contradiction didn't really occur to me until an incident that took place about 10 years or so ago.

I'd gone to find out if I was suitable for laser eye surgery. During the consultation, they put some drops in my eyes that sent my blood pressure through the floor. Within moments I felt woozy and then I was gone – really gone, deep into the land of nod. The next thing I knew, I was being carted off in an ambulance. All very exciting but utterly pointless as it was just a dead faint. Clearly a full, man-sized dose of those drops was a bit too much for me. Still, I rarely take medication of any kind so it's not something I worry about, except for one thing.

There's 11 and a half stone of Mack; nowadays – thanks largely to a fondness for chocolate – there's about seven stone of me. Let's say we both have a headache. I'll take the standard adult dose of two paracetamol because one doesn't usually shift it. Mack will have just one. The thing is, if one's not enough for me, how can it *possibly* be enough for a full-grown man? But it is.

Not all medicines can be split – for example, extended-release tablets. But the propranolol Mack occasionally has to take for a blood pressure spike (one tablet being a normal dose) he carefully cuts into smaller pieces, and that works just fine for him. Same with hay fever pills.

This had me perplexed for years, and I sometimes wondered whether the part-pills worked due to some kind of placebo effect. But now that we've learned so much about his different wiring, sensory sensitivity and the like, it seems to make sense that medication could affect him differently regardless of his comparative size – if he's more sensitive then he shouldn't need as much.

A bit of online research seems to confirm the theory – although there are as many people who are hy*po* as hy*per*sensitive.

😯 **As some autistic people have more sensitivity to medication, it's good to have a diagnosis on their medical file.**

>><<I'd been prescribed 40mg of extended-release propranolol during a particularly difficult time. On my way to work one day, I was decelerating as we approached traffic lights and someone came sailing into the back of me. Normally, I'd be pretty irate – *fuming* in fact – albeit I'd outwardly control my temper well enough. But that day I was so incredibly chilled out I was almost floating. "Oh, it's fine," I told the distraught lady, "Don't worry about it…"

Although her car was pretty much written off, mine wasn't too bad. Even so, I realised the medication must be *way* too strong for me.>>

Mack

20 December

What we probably need to check out next is whether Mack is similarly hypersensitive to natural medicines or the likes of vitamin supplements. We have noticed that when he tries to boost his B12 levels for example, he feels awful after a few days of the recommended dose despite having felt benefits initially. I feel a laboratory experiment coming on.

It's not only the dosage Mack needs to be careful with though, there are some medications he's learned to avoid altogether. When he needs an anti-histamine for example, he has to make sure he chooses a brand that contains cetirizine rather than loratadine, or the palpitations will have him bouncing around like Tigger on a trampoline. He also reacts badly to anxiety meds, some anti-biotics and some anaesthetics.

> <<I had severe toothache at one point – long time ago now – and knew I needed an extraction. It took every ounce of courage I had to get myself to a dentist, never mind tolerate injection after injection after injection which hardly seemed to touch the pain.
>
> The tooth was half out when the impact of the injections hit me. Or perhaps it was the combined effect of my anxiety and the quantity of anaesthetic. Whatever the case, it sent my heart rate *sky* high!
>
> I'm not sure who was having the bigger panic, me or the dentist, but a moment later I'm on the floor and he was ramming me full of glucose trying to get me back. The worst of it was that he couldn't carry on with the extraction. In fact, he had to shove the tooth

> back in and put a stitch in to hold it till it healed. Another nightmare for another day.
>
> If there's a funny side to the story – and I'm not sure there is – it could only be that he got a bigger fright than I did.>>
>
> Mack

There is a suggestion among the autistic community, based on their experiences, that anti-depressants and anti-anxiety medication in particular may work differently in Auties. Many report awful side effects. However, I can't find any research having been done in this area yet, and I know my own, undoubtedly neurotypical friend Chloe – who takes medication for depression – has long complained about side effects. So who knows…

☺ **It's a relief to know Mack's autism diagnosis is now on his medical records, as the doctors can take account of his hypersensitivity to medication as and when he needs treatment in the future.**

Takeaways for Mack
- Mention this hypersensitivity at any medical appointment, as not all doctors are aware that being autistic can have dosage implications for a patient.
- Better still, make sure his medication sensitivity is reflected in his medical notes.

Takeaways for me
- There's no need to worry about this! Phew.

> <<We're lucky that prescriptions are free in Scotland; so it doesn't make any difference to us as individuals whether we have a little or a lot of medication. But it's good to know,

because I only need a little, that I'm saving
other taxpayers a few coffers!>>

Mack

Communication issues

Social communication difficulties

22 December

Before now, I'd have said Mack didn't have any communication difficulties at all. He tells me he's an introvert, but he's way more outgoing than me. And I've never noticed anything out of the ordinary in his exchanges with other people – he seems to get what they mean and they seem to understand him too. Even his Weegie (Glaswegian) sense of humour!

Having said that, when we first met he definitely overdid the eye contact and that was a bit uncomfortable. OK, weird. And after a bit of grilling, he admits to not 'getting' some people. He also admits that he was sent to speech and drama classes (called elocution in those days) from the age of six to help cure a bad stammer. Ten years of that and he could win a Bafta, whatever the part. He reckons that's where he learned to pretend to be just like everyone else – 'masking' as those in the know call it.

> <<It's very hard work – very stressful most of the time – and as a youngster I didn't understand how others seemed to be able to interact so comfortably and easily. Or why some people took umbrage at some of the things I would say when I was simply trying to be helpful. So those classes were a godsend.>>
>
> Mack

I guess I never really believed Mack when he said he was an introvert – all the evidence seemed to say otherwise. Me,

I definitely *am* an introvert. With people I don't know, or don't know well, my conversation tends to be minimal or to the point – although I'd like to think I'm reasonably sociable. Even with people I do know quite well, I can't blabber on for hours on end just for the sake of it – I hate when you reach the point of struggling to find something new to talk about and are left with only 'empty' conversations.

I'm no party animal, and if I'm at a social event I feel obliged to go to, I tend to hang back and clock watch. Mack, on the other hand, will put his best foot forward, genially chatting to anyone and everyone like he's having a ball. So I've always just let him do that. I had absolutely no idea the amount of effort he put into it, which I guess is a tribute to his performance. Had I understood what it was taking out of him, I'd have taken the conch more often – worked harder myself to allow him to hang back more.

As time's gone by, Mack has found himself more and more reluctant to go to such events, and unable to sustain the effort for long. The last party we went to would have been three or four years ago – a summer barbeque to celebrate my sister Marnie's 60th. I thought Mack managed fine, but actually he'd simply adopted an old trick he admits to having used throughout life – he gave himself a job to do, which was to help Marnie's partner Grady man the barbeque.

>>\<\<Having a job to do gives you something to focus on and distracts you from the stress involved in constantly engaging with people, and reading and interacting with them on a purely social or conversational level. Suddenly, it can all be whittled down to simple exchanges about the weather, the

cooking and the food, with the food acting as the focus for both you and the person you're feeding!

It allows you to be visible and take part but at the same time feel slightly protected by the 'uniform' of your function – in this case, co-cook. There's not the same pressure of endless eye contact to correctly read someone, because you're having to concentrate on what you're doing. You have a perfect excuse for any social gaff – because if you're not looking at a person, you can't possibly be reading their body language or expressions. It's like a get-out-of-jail-free card.

I've always found it easier to perform a function. So being treasurer of this, secretary of that, chair of the next thing was the perfect strategy for me. Even being a host, while that's horrendously hard work, is easier than simply being a guest.>>

Mack

23 December

Often, Auties take the things people say literally – which would make expressions like, 'If you do that again, I'll swing for you!' tricky. It's easy to imagine how misunderstandings could arise on both sides of a conversation. Indeed, if you'd like a really good chuckle on that score, try watching Amol Rajan's interview with Autie

Greta Thunberg[3]. In amongst some quick-fire questions towards the end, he asked her, "[Who's the] person you'd most like to meet who's dead?" She puzzled over this for a moment before replying, "I wouldn't want to meet a dead person!" A nano-second later the pair of them dissolved with laughter as light dawned.

Mack doesn't have this problem though. His thing is exaggeration or embellishment. It makes his stories much more entertaining, but you have to guess what *actually* happened.

Oh, and I've just thought of something else that might fall under the umbrella of social communication difficulties – unless it's just my own hang-ups coming to the fore. Quite a lot of the stuff I've been reading mentions that Auties can sometimes be socially inappropriate, and indeed I've often had a fear of Mack saying something totally squirmy in the wrong company!

Here's a random example. Let's say you're taken by a monthly surprise when out and about but don't have a tampon with you. Obviously, you urgently need to find a loo and undertake any damage limitation or mitigation. You could race off leaving Mack in the dust – no explanation – or send him to buy some tampons and meet you back at the loo. The second approach is the more sensible, but it comes with the risk of becoming a hilariously embellished dinner table anecdote. Thankfully, this isn't a real-life example, but I think the danger is genuine. Why? Well, maybe it's absolutely nothing to do with autism and purely that Mack

---

[3] BBC iPlayer (2022), Amol Rajan Interviews: Greta Thunberg. Accessed December 2022 at:
https://www.bbc.co.uk/iplayer/episode/m001d9rg/amol-rajan-interviews-greta-thunberg

and his family are open people who find bodily functions vastly entertaining, while I can be a bit of a prude.

We joke, as a family, about being unable to get through a dinner without the conversation at some point descending to the level of poo. And when this happens, Halle's husband Connor and I just look at each other and roll our eyes while the Mackies virtually fall off their chairs and roll around the floor.

<<Rude!

Having said that, I do recall Halle asking us during lockdown – no doubt on the back of my over-investment in loo roll – how many sheets of loo paper we each used per visit. She was quite insistent, demanding an answer of each of us in turn. The funniest thing was Shonagh's appalled expression and her desperate attempts to avoid answering and to divert the conversation. Yep, that was hilarious!>>

Mack

Glad you think so! What astonishes me is that father and daughter can be so alike and yet Halle insists she's not an Autie. Indeed, she got the lowest score of all of us when we did the AQ50 test online. Don't know how, because I've tried it many, many times to see if I could get my own score down – to no avail. Anyway, back to business…

Sometimes, Mack doesn't seem to know when a conversation is winding down or over – even if he's giving out the winding down signals himself. He'll say something like, "OK, well, I'll let you go now…" but then start off on a completely new topic! Or the other person will pick up their coat and bag, or say, "Well, I'd better be getting on…"

but he'll miss the cue and again begin a whole new thread of conversation. I had just put it down to his love of a natter and have teased him about it many times in the past, but I guess his diagnosis puts this foible in a whole new light.

😲 A social interaction may look and sound casual and comfortable, but it can be exceptionally tiring to keep it up.

> <<It's great having a conversation with Iain [his Autie stonemason pal]. When either of us has had enough, we just stop talking and walk away – no offence taken!>>
>
> Mack

😲 The speech and drama classes have clearly been key to Mack's success in hiding his autism till the seventh decade of his life!

Takeaways for Mack
- Happily, he doesn't need to worry about this one as he pretty much cracked it during childhood.

Takeaways for me
- Be aware how tired he's likely to be after social interactions of any length.
- Maybe we should work a little on the signals for ending conversations.

> <<I realise now that I must have been a very difficult child and – given there wasn't much understanding of autism back in the 60s – I was treated accordingly. This probably made me more nervous and difficult still, and by the age of six I'd not only become scared of my

own shadow but had developed a very bad stammer.

While I was initially sent to the speech and drama classes to cure the stammer, I kept at it, working my way through the grades for 10 years until I received my ALCM diploma. Ironically, achieving this aged 16 meant I'd become the youngest person in the UK then qualified to *teach* speech and drama. (And for a while I did teach others – on a one-to-one basis.)

It was hard-going at times, but those classes helped turn my life around. They gave me the tools to pretend, to 'perform', to appear confident regardless of any trepidation or turmoil inside, and it was such a good feeling to be able to do that. By the time I was 10, not only was my stammer gone, but I'd also learned to use inflection – something I hadn't even realised was missing from my speech. I noticed almost immediately the difference that made though – people suddenly seemed more interested in what I was saying.

One of my fondest memories of that time was when Director of the London College of Music William Lloyd Webber dropped in on the examinations when I was doing my associateship. Meeting him was a big moment for me. And although he was more interested in music than speech and drama, he made some very succinct, helpful and encouraging comments after my set pieces. At that point in my life I hadn't often received any praise or positive feedback, so when it did happen, I truly treasured it.>>

Mack

Listening

27 December

While on the subject of communication… It hadn't really occurred to me before, but Mack doesn't listen very well – he's always interrupting. Interrupting to the point where I often give up halfway through whatever it is I'm trying to tell him. He'll also rant at the TV so that I only get the headline of a news story and can't hear the story itself. Nor can *he*, of course, so he'll often go off at a tangent or ask questions we'd know the answers to if we'd been able to hear.

Worse still, he'll talk over key moments of a film or a TV programme. Imagine, you've invested an hour and a half of your life in a 'who-done-it' or similar, and then you miss the denouement! Ugh! I'd love to say, "*Wheesht!*", but that would be unkind – especially now that I understand he can't help himself.

In a fit of enthusiasm, he'll hammer on with something. I'll tell him, "Slow down" or "Would that not be easier if you let me help?" or "You're overdoing it – take a break", but I'm wasting my breath. Many, many hours later, he'll be exhausted and bemoaning aches and pains or strains. What can you do?

It takes a monumental effort not to say, "Told you so!" If I can't resist it, he'll give me 'the look' and I'll think, now where have I seen reproach like that before? Oh, yes. In the eyes of grandpuppy Haggis when, having produced a perfectly delicious paté from his very own bowels, he's told he's not allowed to eat it.

Our initial research suggested poor listening skills is an Autie 'thing' – that while an Autie's ability to process what they see is 10 times *more* powerful than ours, their ability to process what they hear is 10 times *less* powerful! That's a mind-boggling thought, and it really hit home when we saw images of autistic brains and neurotypical brains lit up alongside each other showing the difference. This not only explains why you can barely get a word in edgeways for Mack's interrupting, it also explains why what you *do* say often doesn't seem to register.

However, while this finding is very true for Mack and the members of his late diagnosis group, it seems it isn't true of all Auties. For example, Number 6's Tom trained and practiced as a psychodynamic counsellor, has trained many staff in third sector organisations he's worked for in 'attentive listening skills', and knows a few autistic counsellors. So, while it may be the case that some Auties – maybe even many – have poor listening skills, quite a lot are pretty good at listening!

Ugh. Getting to grips with autism is a bit like trying to catch a wet fish with your bare hands! Anyway, let's get back to Mack's autistic idiosyncrasies.

My investigations tell me that interrupting is very common with Auties. They tend to listen only to the first few words – or if you're lucky sentences – of what you're saying and guess or assume the rest. And then they'll interrupt and speak over you with their own interpretation or finish your sentence or story for you. Oh, how familiar that sounds!

> <<The truth is that people can often be just a bit slow in translating their thoughts into words. It's like patiently waiting for someone to tell you a joke when you already know the

punchline. Excruciating. I'm not being rude –
I'm being helpful!>>

Mack

Yes, that's what Haggis says when he's digging a hole in your garden.

[Post script:] Interestingly, naturalist Autie Chris Packham echoed Mack's thoughts on this in a recent BBC podcast[4], saying, "…and occasionally people will be explaining things to me and I, I know where they're going. I really, I know what they're going to say. And so I would just speed up the process by jumping to the end of their conversation…"

😲 **If an autistic person interrupts, we can take it as a sign that they're interested or engaged in the conversation. Conversely, if they go quiet, they've probably zoned out and are already thinking about something else!**

This really tickled me, partly because I'm guilty of the zoning out thing too – especially when Mack 'goes off on one' and I've heard it all before. In fact, I spend so much time in the other zone – while still looking as though I'm listening – that I'm sure I must often miss important information. Thankfully, I have a ready-made excuse. I burst an eardrum when I was a student and my hearing in that ear never fully recovered, so I can simply cock my head, innocently say, "Sorry?" and get away with it.

It's not just lack of interest that can cause an Autie to zone out though, it can also happen when they're tired. Mack was

---

[4] BBC Sounds (2023), 1800 Seconds on Autism: Is my dog autistic? With Chris Packham. Accessed May 2023 at:
https://www.bbc.co.uk/programmes/p0fbt754

exhausted at the end of each of the late diagnosis group sessions, and all he had to do was sign in, listen, and make the occasional observation or contribution. And it wasn't just him. According to Mack, you could see the other participants flagging too – zoning in and out with the effort involved – and disappearing off every now and again for some sort of sugar boost. "What, for a two-hour online group meeting?" I hear you say. But it wasn't just any old meeting. These were all people who had been diagnosed well into adulthood and had suddenly found an explanation for the challenges they've spent their whole lives struggling with. That's got to be emotionally draining whether you find meetings easy or not. And it must have been 10 times worse for facilitator Laurent. Sorry, I'm wandering off topic.

Let's get back to the ranting. I can't find anything definitive on this, but I'm thinking that it's at least partly to do with the listening issue. If an Autie gets bored listening after only a few words or sentences, that could explain why I only get the headline before a rant begins. And while I can't find 'scholarly articles' on ranting, I did find quite a few chats among Auties where they said things like, "Ranting allows me to express my emotions," and "Ranting to myself helps me to hear my more confusing thoughts more clearly."

Mack has spent some time ruminating about his ability to listen and it's definitely struck a chord. He tells me he's always learned by reading, by watching and by trying things out rather than by listening to explanations or instructions.

> <<As a kid, I took the TV to bits to figure out how it worked. Dad wandered in, looking forward to watching the football which was due to start shortly, and instead found himself surveying the wreckage! I had barely half an

hour to put it all back together again, with Dad helpfully pacing back and forth. Thankfully, I managed it just in time.

I think I've always preferred to learn that way. I can research something happily for hours on end, and I can deconstruct and fiddle with things for hours too. But listening? My brain can only take so much and it seems to just switch off. I have persistence in spades, but no patience whatsoever.>>

Mack

😐 **I'm not sure whether this new understanding will change anything for Mack or not, but I certainly think it can help *me*.**

Takeaways for Mack
- He wasn't worried about this before, and I'm fairly sure he's not going to start worrying about it now – especially if it's simply the way he's wired and there's nothing he can do about it anyway.

Takeaways for me
- If I want him to know something important, I should probably repeat it two or three times and get some kind of confirmation that it's registered. Better still, write it down!
- There's no point being exasperated if it turns out he hasn't heard – I just need to remember it's a 'thing'. Like when we agree to have fish and chips for dinner and he says later, "What do you fancy for dinner?", or I come home to find he's made something entirely different!

<<I read somewhere that after listening to a lesson or lecture, even neurotypical students have forgotten more than 90% of the information after 14 days. That makes listening an almost pointless exercise.

It certainly supports the proverb 'tell me and I will forget…' – far better to learn by reading (especially if you have a photographic memory that allows you to recall it easily!) or by being shown something and/or simply taking a trial and error approach.>>

Mack

That's quite telling in itself though, isn't it, that Mack's talking in terms of listening being a way of learning? Or *not* learning. He's thinking about information exchange rather than common or garden conversation. Just saying.

Interestingly, Mack's ability to read is a neat counterbalance to his diminished listening skills. I feel honour bound to mention that, lest you feel I've been ribbing him a little ruthlessly here. He can speed read at warp factor eight and has often mentioned that he used to read a book a night as a child. I'd always assumed he was exaggerating, but since discovering hyperlexia, I wonder if I've been doing him wrong!

We first came across the term hyperlexia when reading the blog of OldLady With Autism (another Autie diagnosed very late in life). The American Psychological Association (APA) defines hyperlexia as the development of extremely good reading skills at a very early age, well ahead of word comprehension or cognitive ability. So that's me told then!

28 December

My investigations suggest Auties aren't generally very good at multi-tasking, but again this must vary hugely from person to person. Mack is way better at it than I am. While he seems to be able to switch between tasks without a second thought, I prefer to be left in peace to concentrate on one thing at a time and hate having to juggle several pieces of work at once.

If Mack interrupts me while I'm working to ask if I can do something for him afterwards, I'll try hard to listen without losing my current train of thought. But later, I'll realise that I have little or no recollection of what he asked me to do. I just can't concentrate successfully on the two things at once so have to choose between listening properly and completely losing my place, or rubber-earing him. So how does *he* do it?

> <<Key words. Nobody needs an entire brief, you just need to catch a key word or two.
>
> So if someone says, "Can you please update the X15 test in the monitoring programme with the latest FCA rule changes and send me a copy?" you only need to register 'update X15' because the rest is entirely obvious – a complete waste of words really!>>
>
> Mack

Hmm, I'm not so sure. I agree that I could have worked out what was required purely from 'update X15', but I would have had to listen to the whole waffle to identify that those were the key words. And I couldn't do that at the same time as hanging on to my thread... It's interesting to know that that's how he does it though.

And here's a thing – I've no idea whether it's to do with listening or not, but it's certainly a communication issue of some kind.

Mack is watching TV. I'm sitting beside him reading a book. He'll make a comment to do with whatever he's watching, like, "What does he think he's going to achieve by doing that?" as if I'm watching it too. Although surely he must *know* that I'm not? I'll look up at the TV and try to figure out what he's talking about so that I can make a suitable rejoinder. And then I'll return to my book, albeit I'll have to start the paragraph again.

But within a minute or two, "Oh, that's completely irresponsible showing that on TV – someone's going to end up in hospital!" I look up again, but I've missed the moment. I don't want to be rude, so I show an interest and, once I think it's safe to do so, return to my book. Back to the start of that same paragraph in all likelihood.

And then, "Why don't *we* get one of those?" Just as well I've got the patience of a saint. Unless of course it's *me* who's got the listening problem. Should I be listening more? Probably.

Telepathy

30 December

Mack will call out from a different room and say things like, "Who put this in there?" Unfortunately, I can't see through walls so I have no idea what 'this' is or where 'there' is. But he genuinely thinks I ought to know what he's talking about and gets exasperated when I don't.

I've tried explaining that it would help if he used actual nouns. Why not say, "Who put *my shoes* in *the oven*?" or whatever 'this' and 'there' might be, but he just sighs – like that would be way too much effort.

I can't find much – well, anything really – about this online. Lots about Auties sometimes muddling up their pronouns (me/you), which isn't something Mack's ever done. But nothing about using 'this', 'that' and 'there' instead of meaningful words.

There was a great forum discussion where Auties were agreeing that they often use the wrong word, or even reverse words, when their brains and their mouths aren't quite in sync. But I'm not convinced that's autism-specific. When my own brain's tired or not fully engaged, I often grab the wrong word – usually an alternative or good-enough one, knowing Mack will 'get' it. Only 10 minutes ago when he was wondering what was wrong with the TV, I told him I'd numbed the remote rather than muted it. Anyway, I think *all* of us do more of that as we get older. So no help there.

You know, I think I was probably closer to the mark when I said that he gets exasperated because I don't seem to know what he's talking about. It's not that it would be too much effort to use meaningful words – I'm sure he could find the words if he wanted to – it's that he thinks I'm being difficult. He just can't believe I don't already know what he means.

Following one of his sessions with Number 6, Mack confirmed this is a 'thing' too. Many Auties expect you to know exactly what they're thinking – and worry about it too because they don't necessarily *want* others to be able to see inside their heads!

I don't think Mack worries about *others* having this power of perception. But he does continue to expect it of me!

<<But we were talking about this only yesterday – keep up!>>

Mack

See what I mean? Who remembers *yesterday*?!

Here's my theory. Auties are known for being honest, direct, saying exactly what they think. Telling the white lies of social convention doesn't come naturally to them as it does to neurotypical people. The Auties who have mastered this social skill have learned it the hard way through years and years of social observation and masking. So they *can* say your bum doesn't look big in that, but because it doesn't come naturally or easily, they'll instinctively fear being rumbled, i.e. that despite what they're saying, you know what they're thinking! That would be understandable, wouldn't it?

As I said, just a theory.

😲 When autistic people are in a conversation together, they can pick up from exactly where they left off last time – however long that might have been – with barely a blink.

When I asked Mack if he could think of an example of this, he said, "Yes, of course – Bryson." He's told me about Bryson before, but I've never met him – this was long before my time.

> <<We used to give presentations together on technical compliance matters. It always works better if you have a frequent change of speakers when you're covering a dry topic, it helps keep your audience awake!
>
> Bryson and I had always been on the same wavelength. We could finish each other's thoughts and sentences, and we played off against each other almost as though the presentation were a conversation. We could also cover for each other beautifully so that if there were any hiccups, no one would notice.
>
> I remember starting to choke in the middle of saying something one time and Bryson stepped right in, finishing off what I'd been saying and carrying right on to the next part. And another time, I'd made the mistake of looking around the room and was seized by momentary panic. Again, Bryson stepped smoothly in as though we'd intended to hand over at that point, giving me the time I needed to recover. I'd do the same for him too on occasion.
>
> We didn't use notes, and we didn't rehearse, it just worked. It helped of course that we both knew our stuff inside out.>>
>
> Mack

So maybe it's not about telepathy at all. Lots of studies suggest that communication difficulties happen between Auties and neurotypicals – there are no such problems in an Autie-to-Autie conversation. Turns out this phenomenon is called the double empathy problem.

The double empathy problem is a theory that explains the difficulties people have communicating with someone of a different neurotype. Here's how the National Autistic Society describes it:

"Simply put, the theory suggests that when people with very different experiences of the world interact with one another, they will struggle to empathise with each other. This is likely to be exacerbated through differences in language use and comprehension... This theory would also suggest that those with similar experiences are more likely to form connections and a level of understanding."[5]

So maybe Mack should've married Bryson rather than me! Presumably, he wouldn't have needed to ask *him* why he'd put the shoes in the oven.

Here are just a few examples of where a little telepathy – or a little more empathy! – between us would be particularly helpful.

I'm getting myself a drink so yell through to Mack: "Would you like a full-fat coke?" anticipating that this would be his likely preference. Clearly, I'm expecting an affirmative response. Like, "Yes, please." But what I get instead is, "Well, my tummy's been upset all morning." Ugh. What does that mean? I wait, in the hope of clarification. It

---

[5] National Autistic Society (2018), The double empathy problem. Accessed December 2022 at:
https://www.autism.org.uk/advice-and-guidance/professional-practice/double-empathy

doesn't come, so I have to try and figure it out. Have *you* got it yet? Full marks for a 'yes', and a bonus point if you reckon you know why. It's because he thinks the bubbles might help his tummy! Sadly, I'd never have got that one.

What's gone wrong here is that he's failed to convey the connection between his answer and my question, because he thinks it's obvious – or that I should already know or be able to work it out. I'd like to say I'm getting better at deducing what he means, but the truth is that my brain frequently hurts trying to figure out the relationship between his responses and my questions!

My head's in the fridge now, checking to see what there might be to eat. "What do you want for lunch?" I ask him, "Soup? A ham sandwich? Toasted cheese?" These are pretty much the only options. "Em…" he says. "…before I die of hypothermia, preferably…" He gives me a look. "I could do with more protein, and maybe more fibre today," he tells me, thinking he's given me the answer I need. Of course, he'll know which of these options fits that bill best, but again fails to relay it and I confess my nutritional expertise isn't what it might be. Should I google or guess, do you think?

We're watching some antique-type programme and someone with a Weegie accent is talking about the stately home they're filming at. "Where's that?" I ask Mack. "Glasgow," he says. "Yes, but where *is* it?" I repeat, realising he's missed my meaning. "Just round from where Dad used to live." "No, I mean… what's the *building*?!" Of course, this one's entirely my fault because, for once, he gave exactly the right answer in a nutshell. This time, it was *me* expecting *him* to be telepathic!

Sometimes, it's hard work being me (to pinch one of his own lines!)

😕 **We're both going to need to put a little more effort into this.**

Takeaways for Mack
- Forget sci-fi, telepathy isn't actually a thing.
- Use a few nouns to give his listener a fighting chance of figuring out what he's on about.
- Try giving a specific answer to a specific question from time to time. A 'yes' or a 'no' would be really good!

Takeaways for me
- Work on my empathy!
- Patience is a virtue.

Interaction and anxiety

General anxiety

2 January

Mack once said to me, "How would you describe me, in only one word?" That kind of test always flummoxes me – too many options. Plus, what answer does he expect or actually want to hear, and would whatever I come up with be tactful?! His own answer surprised me a bit: *anxious* he said.

He doesn't come over that way. He comes over as confident, outgoing, affable… and he generally *looks* relaxed. (Guess I have a bad habit of taking everyone and everything at face value.)

Now that I understand about sensory sensitivity, I can see how you might be anxious when out and about – the fear of sensory overload and the resulting panic attacks or even meltdowns if you find yourself in an overload situation you can't escape from. That would be horrible. Frightening even.

I came home from work one day 10, maybe 15 years ago, to find Mack looking seriously washed out. He'd spent most of the day in hospital after having called himself an ambulance, utterly convinced he was having a heart attack. That was his first full-on panic attack.

> <<The least thing can trigger a panic attack really.
>
> It's like… you're in a store, and everything's fine. Suddenly it gets busy, noisy – the people, the tannoy, the echo – you start to get tense and that brings on some vision

>disturbance. You feel lightheaded, stressed, and have a feeling of dread, of being trapped. Your heart starts racing, palpitations begin, you feel hot, your hands are sweaty – mouth dry, can't breathe, can't think straight – you're overcome with an irrational fear – panic – the need to escape – to just get out, get out, get out...!

And afterwards, well, you're just *wiped* by this over*whelming* fatigue.>>

Mack

This may sound odd, but I was very impressed that he'd had the gumption to call an ambulance. To me, that was the stuff of TV shows rather than real life – as though an ambulance was some imaginative sci-fi concept like the Tardis or the starship Enterprise.

A decade earlier, I'd singularly failed to even *think* of calling 999 when I found myself increasingly struggling to breathe one evening. I just puffed away on my inhaler, hoping that would help. Knowing the nearest doctor's practice wouldn't be open till 8am, I built myself a wee nest in an armchair thinking I'd be able to sleep sitting up that night. But actually, I was too scared to fall asleep in case my breathing stopped altogether – every breath was such an effort.

My mother swooped in to the rescue next morning, rushing me to the hospital where I spent the next eight nights. Even then I felt a bit of a fraud, until the consultant and a bunch of medical students stood chatting around my bed about how many people die of asthma each year and how lucky I was. I didn't feel lucky – I felt like a zoo exhibit – but it was only then that I wondered whether I ought to have called for help earlier. So maybe there's an upside to being a worrier like Mack – you're much more likely to seek help while there's still time!

It's not only the fear of sensory overload that causes anxiety though. It seems that almost every Autie I've read about – and I've been doing lots of reading! – was relentlessly bullied as a child because they were 'different', and that must seriously dent your self-confidence. All Mack's years of speech and drama classes taught him how to present a confident picture to the world, but maybe the anxiety pummelled into you through your childhood never leaves you, I don't know.

Fellow traveller Sabrina – whose husband and elder child are both autistic and have ADHD (attention deficit hyperactivity disorder) – observed that when you live in a constantly anxious state, you desensitise to it and then can't work out when to really respond. When I mentioned this to Mack, he agreed.

<<If you're already in a state of high alert, you're likely to respond the same way no matter how big or small the challenge. For example, if you've wound yourself up to high doh to face a medical appointment and you're given bad news, you don't know how to alter or escalate your response because you're already on the ceiling.>>

Mack

😮 **What is clear – regardless of any root cause – is that for most, anxiety is a huge part of autism.**

There were some gems about this in the Guardian article[6] I mentioned earlier when talking about interoception. It said that people with anxiety pay close attention to their body signals, but don't necessarily *read* them correctly. For example, they might believe a small change in heart rate is much bigger than it really is, leading to a sense of panic. It also talked about growing evidence that signals from our internal organs to our brain play a key part in regulating our emotions and warding off anxiety and depression. Which supports the idea that learning to read those signals correctly could make a real difference to an Autie's general anxiety levels.

During particularly hard times in Mack's life, he's considered anxiety meds and tried them a couple of times. However, he reacted badly to them and gave up because the side effects were worse than the anxiety. Instead, he tried to reorganise his life to reduce stressors as much as he could.

> <<I think it was the shingles that really knocked me for six. The anti-virals left me with no energy and a foggy brain, and I found that for long enough I simply couldn't function. Even my memory was failing me, and trying to carry on as before just wasn't an option.
>
> So I reduced my workload by appointing one of the guys as managing director, I stopped doing face-to-face client work so that I wouldn't have to travel anymore, and I

---

[6] The Guardian (2021), Interoception: the hidden sense that shapes wellbeing. Accessed December 2022 at:
https://www.theguardian.com/science/2021/aug/15/the-hidden-sense-shaping-your-wellbeing-interoception

reduced the days and hours I spent in the office in favour of working from home more.

It was incredibly hard relinquishing that much control, but at that point I felt I had no choice. And even though I did gradually recover from the shingles, my general anxiety levels remained higher than before and I found I simply couldn't face returning to the full-on stresses of pre-shingles work life.>>

Mack

3 January

Getting work stress levels under control was a huge step forward, but we can't avoid everything in life that's stressful, so Mack has still needed a few tricks up his sleeve to manage day-to-day challenges. A trip to the dentist's for example.

Thanks to the Edinburgh Special Care Dentistry team, Mack now has a great dentist who explains exactly what she's going to do and how long it will take, and does a countdown of each step for him. He finds the counting thing enormously helpful – especially when he can also see a clock – and occasionally tries that same trick to help him navigate other stressful events.

The online group sessions with Number 6 gave Mack lots of other useful tips to help manage general anxiety. Let's say you're going to be giving an important presentation or speech. You might spend a few days preparing for it and maybe getting a little nervous about it if you're not a seasoned performer. Your nerves increase the closer you get to the event, and you're on an adrenalin high while you're actually speaking. A rush of adrenalin is the body's natural response when you're scared, angry or excited; it makes your heart beat faster and prepares your body to react to danger. Afterwards, your adrenalin levels drop off as you begin to relax, which is when the tiredness is likely to hit you. Again, your body's natural response.

For an Autie it's the same, but significantly amplified because the adrenalin rush is higher, and don't forget they have all their sensory sensitivity challenges to cope with too. The Autie will be so exhausted afterwards it may take them *days* to fully recover.

Number 6's advice is pacing and resting. I don't mean 'striding out' pacing – though Mack does plenty of that! – I mean he needs to pace himself such that eventful days are preceded and followed by restful ones. Even each day should be punctuated with respites.

This isn't easy for working Auties because there are few opportunities in the neurotypical world to relax and recuperate. It wouldn't occur to most people, employers or colleagues, that anyone would need the level of rest an autistic person needs – after all, until you begin to explore and understand autism, how would you know?

Even after 20-odd years of knowing Mack, I didn't appreciate the mental energy it took for him to mask and get through each day. No wonder he eventually ceased to function.

😐 **The autistic mind needs time to prepare for something as well as recovery time afterwards.**

Takeaways for Mack
- Schedule sufficient rest time before and after any stressful event to prepare for and recover from it.
- No more scoffing 'mindfulness' and relaxation exercises, as they could make the world of difference!

- Count, breathe, listen to music and take naps – or at least time-outs.

Takeaways for me
- No more springing surprises on him. Turns out it's a mistake to think I'm sparing him anxiety by not telling him visitors are on their way!
- Don't plan more than one 'event' in a day if at all possible.

> <<Until my late 50s, I always managed to get by in terms of dealing with day-to-day stressors. For work-related things for example, I'd be wearing business attire – to me, a suit of armour which I drew strength from. For social things, I'd play the part I believed people expected of me. I literally performed. But it was exhausting.
>
> When I 'hit the wall', it felt as though my strength had dissipated, and I simply couldn't do the things I used to do. When I tried, often my heart rate and blood pressure would skyrocket, and I'd have to take something to bring them back down again. It was a very reactive approach, not a solution. That's why I eventually decided to give the anxiety meds a try (for the second time), but sadly that didn't work out – in fact, it nearly hospitalised me!
>
> Now that I understand autism, what I've been experiencing makes so much more sense. And by applying a lot of the ideas I've gleaned from the sessions with Number 6, I should be able to take a much more proactive approach

to managing my day-to-day life, without putting such a strain on my body and soul!>>

Mack

Social anxiety

5 January

Mack is a social person – more so than me. He'll stop and natter to people – often for ages – when I'd just have smiled and said hello in passing. He'll say he's happy in his own company but can't go longer than a few hours without picking up the phone to chat to someone. And he'll feel forlorn if I go to meet friends or family without him – he *wants* to see them but the thought of going into an environment he can't control comes with a creeping anxiety.

Social anxiety seems to be just another layer on top of the general stuff. It seems odd to me that an ostensibly social person would feel this, but it's a 'thing'. I wonder whether it's caused or made worse for Auties by their life experiences though.

As I mentioned earlier, virtually every Autie I've heard or read about was bullied as a child. They've learned over the years how to mask and fit in, but when they were children their differences will have been much more obvious.

I never knew Mack as a child, but I do know he had a bad stammer when he was little. I know he used to correct his primary school teachers when they made mistakes, which must have made him very unpopular with staff and pupils alike. Nobody likes a know-it-all! And I know the bullying between the ages of 10 and 13/14 was beyond horrific and only stopped when he joined the army cadets and learned unarmed combat and how to shoot. It must leave its mark on you and make you innately wary of people.

> <<Joining the cadets was a game-changer for me. The regime was clear, simple, structured,

orderly – everyone knew and followed the 'rules'. At the same time, you felt both part of something and empowered, stronger, safer, more confident. I learned not just *how* to defend myself but that I actually *could*!

It took a while though, and in the meantime, I'd also found two other safe harbours to help me through my high school days.

Becoming a school librarian gave me the opportunity to escape the dangers of the playground during breaks – the library was a place of safety, a sanctuary. And music was my other great escape. You could lose yourself in a whole other world that provided respite for the soul and was challenging and satisfying at the same time. If ever there was a time when I could say I felt 'happy', it would have been when playing music – particularly performing in concerts with the orchestra.>>

Mack

6 January

Mack describes a 'hierarchy of anxiety'. He lives his life in a state of alert even when he's at home, in a safe environment, constantly scanning without necessarily even being aware of it.

Then, when he's out and about, his general anxiety levels are raised with the change in environment and having to process a tonne of sensory information.

Social anxiety is the next level, bringing with it the need to interact – to talk, to look and behave just like everyone else, to 'perform'. So, even when you *want* to be with people, to enjoy their company and chat and have fun, it's just not that easy.

If and when it all gets too much, well that's when you get meltdown.

> <<Looking back, I suppose I didn't help myself. I always had to try and excel, pushing the boat ever further into the choppy waters of Autiedom.
>
> For the kids' birthdays when they were young, on top of presents, balloons and cakes, I used to invite my parents to join us and I'd lay on a five-course gourmet dinner. I created a ridiculous amount of work for myself with the planning, shopping, preparing, cooking, entertaining and clearing up, all within the short amount of time I had with the kids.
>
> Time spent with them was special and I'd push myself to extremes to try and make it special for them too. And to prove myself to my parents – even as an adult I still longed for some kind of approval.
>
> The moral of the story is not to heap extra, unnecessary anxiety on myself. After all, no one expects Masterchef – and indeed the effort's wasted on some!>>
>
> Mack

When I see Mack acting the clown in social gatherings – such as for the kids' birthdays even nowadays – I know the effort this takes and now watch out for the severe low that follows from the exhaustion.

😮 **Social interactions are hard work as autistic people have to concentrate on so much to sustain a conversation – making eye contact, reading expressions and body language, interpreting hints, implications and 'hidden' meanings.**

Social interaction must be harder still for introverts – as Mack claims to be despite how well he performs – and for Auties who take things literally, as some have a tendency to do. They'll be anxious not to make a mistake and come over as gauche or worse, or inadvertently give offence.

I've only met one or two people in my life I found hard to read and interact with. I'm thinking of one lady in particular; she would tell me a story and end it on a triumphant note as if to say, "What do you think of that?!" A response was clearly required, and I would feel momentary panic because I had absolutely no idea whether the right answer was, "Oh, how awful!" or "Oh, that's amazing!" And I'm a neurotypical person (well, maybe on the cusp if there is such a thing!).

The only clues were in her personality, by which I mean I'd have to guess how *she'd* feel about it, but I just didn't know or understand her well enough to gauge that. It meant I had to really concentrate on her stories, looking for clues, so as not to be caught out. So I can see that it would be hard-going for an Autie if they found many conversations to be like that.

>> <<Despite my speech and drama training, I always found giving presentations and lectures hard. One of the tricks I tried was to focus on only one person in the audience and make eye contact with them – the thought process being that speaking to one person and 'blocking out' all the others would be less

stressful yet still give me the feedback I needed.

Of course, all I was thinking about was myself, not the message I might inadvertently be giving out. Suffice to say my boss at the time was not impressed when afterwards I received some 'fan mail' with a pair of knickers enclosed!>>

Mack

I guess had he been a single man on the pull, this could be considered an upside of his social anxiety!

☹ **While social anxiety is clearly a 'thing', and at the top of the hierarchy, it looks as though there could at least be ways to reduce *overall* anxiety levels to avoid reaching meltdown.**

Takeaways for Mack
- Rest in advance of social events to build energy reserves, and take time to recover afterwards.
- Take time-outs during events.
- Keep to hand earplugs – the kind that muffle background noise while keeping conversation clear.

Takeaways for me
- Increase the number of social events that take place at home or in another familiar environment rather than somewhere new if possible. This should reduce the risk of sensory overload due to non-social factors.

7 January

The whole topic of eye contact fascinates me. It's not something I'm even aware of usually – although sometimes it does occur to me that I'm looking more generally at someone's face rather than their eyes.

Mack tells me eye contact is something he used to do a lot in his professional life – particularly during compliance interrogations. I wouldn't have liked to have been on the other side of that desk, as I can confirm there's nothing more unsettling than having a Weegie stare right through you, unblinkingly, for any length of time. And I'm not sure that, as an Autie, he should even be able to do that, but I guess that's the benefit of all those speech and drama classes.

When I realised eye contact was an issue for Auties (probably first from watching *Mercury Rising*!), it made me think about animals, because I'm certain that some wildlife documentary or other had warned me that you should never look a grizzly bear in the eye or it would attack you. Fortunately, there aren't very many of those wandering the streets of Scotland.

But it's not just grizzly bears. Many species perceive eye contact as a threat. Most animals just don't do direct eye contact as it makes them uncomfortable or anxious – particularly flighty rather than fighty types, such as horses or deer. So, given we're animals too, what's happening here with the Autie brain isn't unusual. Especially given they're generally kind and gentle just like horses and deer. Perhaps they instinctively perceive the average neurotypical person to be a grizzly bear! Which, given their early life experiences, is probably fair.

Turns out the answer is much more scientific than that. Positively dull in fact. There's a bit of the brain – the subcortical system – that responds to eye contact and, in Auties, it's oversensitive which causes discomfort or stress.

At Number 6, they talk about eye contact as a sensory processing issue. If an autistic person is trying to articulate something or needs to think carefully about what they're saying to another person, it's hard to maintain eye contact because there are too many other distractions in front of them – the other person's facial expression, their body language, their clothing, whatever might be going on behind them. It's much easier to articulate when your focus is fixed on something that isn't moving – the floor or the ceiling for example. Yep, I can relate to that.

Meltdowns

9 January

Meltdowns happen as a result of anxiety and way too much adrenalin, or plain sensory overload. I've not always been great at seeing these coming in the past, but I have a much better idea of what to look out for now. A deterioration in Mack's language is usually a good clue that he's reaching the end of his rope! When the 'f' word in particular slips out, I know to give him space and rescue any precious breakables from within his immediate reach.

While reading the fascinating by-Auties-for-Auties book *Been There. Done That. Try This!*[7], I came across a piece by Richard Maguire who described three ways a meltdown can manifest itself, for him.

😳 **The first type of meltdown is as an explosion of violence, the second running away, and the third becoming totally passive and playing dead**.

This seems to fit neatly with what Number 6 termed fight, flight or freeze, which makes perfect sense.

For Mack, the explosive or fight response is extremely rare; I've only witnessed it twice. On the first occasion, 20-odd years ago, he'd just come off an extremely fraught and emotionally charged phone call, and the phone itself took the full impact of his frustration and rage. It ended its life as a whimpering pile of broken plastic and components, and he was left with no (landline) phone.

---

[7] Attwood, T; Evans, CR; Lesko, A (edited by) (2014), Been There. Done That. Try This! An Aspie's Guide to Life on Earth. London and Philadelphia, Jessica Kingsley Publishers.

The second occasion was only last year when he opened the study window and hurled the printer full-force down onto the patio below. And we were left with no printer. Given that the printer was the objectionable blighter that had triggered this meltdown in the first place, it was probably no real loss. But I was a little stunned. I knew he was getting exasperated with it, but hadn't appreciated we were approaching DEFCON 1 till it was too late.

Actually, omelettes can spark a similar reaction. I'd forgotten about them, but once or twice when an omelette's gone wrong in the making, the pan has found itself bouncing off the floor, splattering the entire kitchen in egg. Scrambled egg is definitely a safer option!

The running away or flight response is much more common, and perfectly describes how Mack reacts to sensory overload – escaping from crowds, stores or restaurants at the speed of light. I didn't realise that this could qualify as a meltdown – I'd always thought of these as migraine attacks and/or panic attacks.

But it was the third of Richard's descriptions that rang a particular bell with me, as it suddenly shed light on a previously inexplicable incident that happened about 20 years back. The two of us were in an airport with my sister Marnie, and my niece and her friend, ready to check in for a return flight from Spain. We looked at the monitor to find out which desk to go to, only to read that the gate was closed and the flight was about to depart.

I was confused. Marnie freaked out. And Mack sat quietly down on his suitcase and froze – or, as described by Richard, became totally passive and played dead. That actually distracted me a little from the unfolding drama, as I would have expected Mack to have responded by either taking control (more likely as the most-seasoned flyer amongst us) or by joining the panic. It's the only time I've seen this happen to him and this new understanding of the incident has been a revelation to me!

(It turned out to be a mistake by the way. The gate hadn't even opened for check-in yet, although it took us a good 20 minutes of manic headless-chicken activity to reach this conclusion.)

😏 **If and when Mack's language begins to turn blue, I know stress is building – it's often the first sign that a meltdown's on the way.**

> <<I know people mean well when they say things like, 'don't worry', 'relax/chill out' or 'it'll all be OK', but it's *really* not helpful. In fact, it just adds to what's already a stressful situation.>>
>
> Mack

I think there's also some confusion around much of the terminology we're using while investigating autism though. When I read terms I'm familiar with from my everyday vocabulary, I attribute their everyday meanings to them. So, to me, a meltdown is a description of what happens to someone who becomes overwhelmingly upset – the explosive reaction being one example. And I'd expect breaking down to be another, although that's not listed in the above descriptions. Does this mean that a breakdown of inconsolable and uncontrollable weeping of the I-can't-go-on variety *isn't* a meltdown? To add to my confusion, some people call the playing dead meltdown a shutdown.

It seems to me that we'll perhaps need to wait another few years for definitions to iron themselves out as research and understanding of autism develops further. In the meantime,

I'm going to have to revisit some of my understandings in case there are other layman's terms used in Autie world that may have taken on slightly different meanings. What a minefield. But I'm digressing again.

Essentially, this whole journey is about finding ways to reduce overload and anxiety so that it doesn't reach melting point. All the tricks we've discovered so far – like breathing, counting, timeout, etc – can help. And the strategy that works best will depend on each situation.

Takeaways for Mack
- If sensory overload precautions aren't working, get away from the offending environment.
- If he can't escape the situation, adopt all possible calming strategies.

Takeaways for me
- Avoid giving empty assurances. Instead, try to talk him down with some context or perspective.
- So, rather than reassuring him he won't get killed crossing the road, remind him there's only a one in 240 lifetime risk of that happening. Which he could reduce by following the 'kerb drill'. (Anyone else remember the Tufty Club? – Yep, showing my age!)

I think that last point's quite important – *facts* matter to an Autie.

I've been looking at all sorts of information online about different ways to combat anxiety. The general consensus is that you should try to counter negative thoughts with positive ones. For example, if you're worried that you won't wake up after a general anaesthetic (a favourite current worry of Mack's), you should remind yourself that the risk is very low, that you're pretty healthy, and that the point of the procedure is to improve your health so it'll all be worth it in the end.

'Very low' is no good to an Autie though – certainly not to Mack. He needs to know that, according to the NHS, if you're healthy and having non-emergency surgery, the risk of dying is one in 100,000 general anaesthetics. Only on knowing that would Mack be able to even *hear* the rest of the sentence!

Even then, he'll perceive that as *your* risk, not his. Auties seem to live their lives by Sod's Law – anything that can go wrong will go wrong, usually in the worst possible way. While he'll be pleased to hear about the 99,999 folk who will be just fine, he'll still worry about that one person who won't be and fear that it's just as likely to be him as anyone else. And, suddenly, that one in 100,000 chance sounds more like 50:50!

Auties aren't the only people who can have meltdowns of course. The question is, whether you're an Autie or not, is there an upside to a meltdown?

You could argue that a potential upside of the fight/explosive type is that it allows you to vent, releasing built-up tension. So long as you direct your explosion on expendable items, that sounds like it could be good therapy!

An upside of the flight/run-away meltdown…? Not sure about this one, although getting away from the offending situation or environment has to be better than enduring a level of stress that's going to bring on a full-blown panic attack.

When mulling over the freeze/passive-play-dead – or shutdown – type of meltdown, I found vague memories of WW2 spy stories sprang to mind. Didn't they used to try dissociating as a way of enduring Nazi interrogation or torture? A little bit of googling tells me that dissociation is when you detach yourself from your body, emotions or environment, and that it can be an involuntary way of coping with acute stress you can't physically escape from. OK, a ham-fisted interpretation I admit. But it sounds very much like the freeze meltdown to me.

<<I wonder whether my autism – or specifically the reaction of shutting down under extreme stress – actually helped me through some of my worst experiences in life…>>

Mack

Self-worth

11 January

Many people seem to struggle with impending retirement. Part of it is wondering what they'll do with all their free time, but it seems to me that – with men in particular – they also fear a loss of identity and status. Who are they if they're no longer whatever it is they've been in their job or achieved in their career?

Mack has spent his life trying to prove himself, trying to be the very best he could be at whatever he tried to do, in search of some kind of recognition or approval. And to prove everyone wrong.

If you were that 'difficult' or 'odd' child, always being admonished, punished and persecuted, this is an understandable – admirable – response. And it served him well. By using all the tricks he learned in his 10 years of speech and drama training, he presented to the world a confident, capable, professional façade that allowed him to develop a very successful career. Albeit it was extremely exhausting.

It was war reporter Fergal Keane who spoke these words when talking about what had driven *him* in the career that nearly destroyed him: "We all want to be told that we're worthwhile… but I wanted it more than most. And that's a consequence of course of not feeling that as a child."[8] While their circumstances and experiences were different, it could just as easily have been Mack who said that.

---

[8] BBC iPlayer (2022), Fergal Keane: Living with PTSD. Accessed January 2023 at:
https://www.bbc.co.uk/programmes/m0017795

I guess, if you've never had praise and encouragement to instil self-belief and give you a sense of self-worth as a person, work-related accomplishments would be a great substitute. But when you come to the end of that road, your career is over and you see all you are only in terms of what you've done or achieved in your working life, who or what are you now?

<<I was driven from a young age. At six or seven, I filled a bag from our fruit bowl and went round the neighbours selling fruit. I also tried to sell pages from Dad's Glasgow Herald. Luckily, many of the neighbours were business people and they were tickled by my entrepreneurial spirit.

From 13, I worked Saturdays in a shoe shop for a wonderful man who taught me the basics of business (as well as respect for others and how to be a decent human being). And as soon as I passed my driving test, he let me borrow his car and encouraged me to sell stock at Ingliston market every Sunday, keeping the majority of the profit. He was the first person I ever remember who praised and encouraged me, and I miss him to this day.

It was 23 years later before I finally set up my own business and, to be honest, that was more due to circumstance than choice at the time, as my self-confidence was at a very low ebb following the break-up of my first marriage and a bad job move. Somehow, thanks to my speech and drama training and suit of armour, things worked out – despite a rocky start, the company was successful and built up a rock-solid reputation. And I'd proved to myself that I could do it.

Since selling, I've continued to consult – but I can't put retirement off any longer. It's a little like looking into an abyss...>>

Mack

12 January

Whenever Mack's feeling depressed, he'll be overcome with a sense of failure and worthlessness that mystifies me because I believe he's made a pretty good fist of his life. Especially when you consider how much he must have struggled through his childhood and how the odds have been stacked against him.

😮 **The effects of childhood experiences such as abuse, rejection, trauma and bullying can lead to feelings of worthlessness that last deep into adulthood.**

Feelings of being unworthy, 'less than' or underachievement can bleed into every aspect of your life, adding to social anxiety. To counter these feelings, I try to remind Mack of some of the things he *has* achieved.

When I first met him, he was listed in the business version of Who's Who and had such a good reputation that he was invited to speak at all sorts of places, including Harvard University and the Federal Reserve Bank. He was even awarded an honorary doctorate from one of the US universities for his work – though he was too embarrassed to own this!

On top of his day job, he was a president of the Securities Institute in Scotland, having been involved in building up the Scottish region from scratch, and was elected by the membership to the UK Board of the Institute. He was also a verifier of investment regulation examinations for the Chartered Institute of Bankers in Scotland.

Given that 20% of start-up businesses fail in their first year and 60% don't make it past three years, he should feel proud of having set up and run his own business for 18 years, surviving both 9/11 and the financial crash of 2007-2008. During this time, he was given a lifetime achievement award for compliance services and is still held in high regard by the industry today.

However, I fear Mack's expectations of himself had been sky high, and maybe nothing short of the achievements of Albert Einstein or Steve Jobs would have been enough.

> <<You try to do the best you can and make the most of what you've got, but it feels as though nothing is ever enough. One upside is that autism clearly gave me some gifts that I was able to use to my advantage in my line of work, but now that work is behind me… I'm lost.>>
>
> Mack

In her book *Taking off the Mask*[9], author Dr Belcher talked about typical 'thinking errors' that Auties are prone to – fascinating stuff that helps explain why Mack's feelings of self-worth remain low despite all my efforts to point out why he ought to feel positive about himself. The way Auties think means they tend to:

- Ignore the positives – as they're too busy worrying about the negatives.

---

[9] Belcher, Dr HL (2022) Taking off the Mask. London, Jessica Kingsley Publishers.

- Blow things out of proportion – making small things feel huge.
- Predict the worst – believing that if something could go wrong, it will.
- Believe people are thinking badly of them – probably because they don't read others very well.
- Label things negatively – so they think badly about themselves because of the least little thing.
- Set the bar too high – thinking they always have to be perfect, otherwise they're worthless.
- Blame themselves for things – even if there's no evidence they've done anything wrong.
- Take their feelings as facts – so if they fear they've messed up, it must be true.
- Wallow in 'should haves' if things don't go quite right – even though no one is gifted with perfect foresight.

The NHS[10] talks about the link between low self-esteem and social anxiety. They say that if you have low self-esteem or confidence, you may well hide away from social situations, stop trying new things, and avoid things you find challenging. That applies to anyone, not just an Autie. And the trouble is, this reinforces your underlying doubts and fears.

The two most obvious things that can promote feelings of self-worth are to experience unconditional love, respect, and appreciation – largely missing from Mack's early life – or to experience success. The latter explains Mack's driving ambition through adulthood. But now that he's retiring, it

---

[10] NHS (2020), Raising low self-esteem. Accessed January 2023 at:
https://www.nhs.uk/mental-health/self-help/tips-and-support/raise-low-self-esteem

seems that he sees opportunities for success as having come to an end.

Somehow, we need to move his mind to a healthier place. To stop placing value on money, reputation, accolades or social or professional status and instead think about things that really matter. How kind he is, how generous, how well he treats people. Maybe it would help if he listed a number of the people he loves and respects and then asked himself what the qualities are in those people that he values. It's highly unlikely that wealth or earth-shattering achievements would come into it.

And given that – despite his professional achievements – he still feels unfulfilled, it would do no harm to look at his non-professional achievements and acts of kindness over the years to help fight off the failure monster and boost his self-esteem.

For example, Mack was an instrumental member of his local Rotaract Club from the age of 18, helping raise many thousands of pounds for charities in the local community. He fondly remembers their projects to provide baby monitors for Yorkhill Hospital to help prevent cot deaths, Christmas boxes for struggling pensioners, and little cars ('row cars') to help disabled children get around on their own.

> <<I was district treasurer at the time of the row cars project and we managed to raise £50,000 which, in the late 1970s, was a lot of money! We got 10 of the cars for our own club which went to local kids, and I had the pleasure of seeing them all lined up in their

> little row cars showing their new-found independence – big smiles all round!>>

Mack

From the Rotaract, Mack joined the Round Table, a similar organisation for 28 to 40-year-olds which had the same business and charitable objectives. They did all sorts of things from organising helicopter rides for profoundly disabled kids to helping the local fire service with injured veterans.

> <<One of the kids in the helicopter had Down's syndrome. He was so excited by the experience – having never been out of his house except for medical appointments before – that he took to screaming, "Aghhhhhhhhhh!" when the helicopter was going up, and "Wheeeeeeeee!" when coming down. We could hear him from 100 feet below, and he wouldn't let anyone else have a go! Seeing these kids happy was the best thing ever.>>

Mack

Mack also served on the Children's Panel for three years, driven by a desire to help kids avoid the dangers of physical and sexual abuse, drugs and family discord. The role of a panel member is to listen and make legal decisions with and for infants, children and young people in children's hearings. Emotionally, this was an exceptionally draining experience. But one which will have undoubtedly helped make a positive difference to countless children's lives.

😊 **Building stronger feelings of self-worth can boost self-esteem and reduce social anxiety.**

Takeaways for Mack
- Identify and challenge negative beliefs about himself.
- Focus on the things he *has* achieved, and recognise the things he's good at.
- Consider getting involved with charity work again.

Takeaways for me
- Demonstrate my own unconditional love, respect and appreciation of him more often – I suspect I'm rubbish at that. Scotch that – I *know* I'm rubbish at that!

Depression

15 January

I found it quite distressing to learn that Auties are very prone to depression and suicidal thoughts.

I know there have been dark times in Mack's life, but I'm not sure how much of the resulting depression was due to autism and how much to his experiences, because I think some of the things he's been through would have had the same effect on most people.

For example, he described to me – way back when we first met – the absolute desolation he'd felt at leaving his children behind when his first marriage broke up. For a short while, he saw the world through the bottom of a glass, and I know he considered checking out, courtesy of a fast car. What stopped him was seeing his kids' faces in his mind's eye at the last moment and he just couldn't do it. Thankfully.

I believe he's only felt *that* bad a few times, but he's certainly battled with depression on and off all the time I've known him. Perhaps always. It's so sad to know that about someone who is so talented, smart, caring and otherwise full of fun.

😧 **Autistic people make up 1% of the population but 11% of suicides, and up to 66% of autistic adults have considered suicide.**[11]

---

[11] Royal College of Psychiatrists (2021), Suicide and Autism, a National Crisis. Accessed January 2023 at:
https://www.rcpsych.ac.uk/docs/default-source/improving-care/nccmh/suicide-prevention/workshops-(wave-4)/wave-4-workshop-2/suicide-and-autism---slides.pdf?sfvrsn=bf3e0113_2

While I was researching this topic, I came across a Guardian article called *'All my life suddenly made sense': how it feels to be diagnosed with autism late in life*.[12] In it, Simon Baron-Cohen, who works in the field of autism research, is quoted as saying, "To my mind, [suicidal feelings are] nothing to do with autism… These are secondary mental health problems. You came into the world with autism, and the way the world reacted, or didn't react, to you has led to a second problem, which is depression."

It's vexing, to say the least, that the burden of depression – on top of the challenges autism alone presents – is so unnecessary.

During the darkest times, Mack has turned to the Samaritans, a charity that provides emotional support to anyone in emotional distress or at risk of suicide.

> <<I know when things get that bad you're supposed to talk to someone – but it's very hard to put a burden like that on someone else. The last thing I want to do is drag my wife or kids down with me, and so it bottles up to the point where it becomes utterly unbearable.
>
> That's why I first called the Samaritans. I'm not sure what I expected, and it wasn't an easy call, but it was certainly easier talking to a stranger – a non-judgemental person you'll never meet or even speak to again – than

---

[12] The Guardian (2016), 'All my life suddenly made sense': how it feels to be diagnosed with autism late in life. Accessed January 2023 at:
https://www.theguardian.com/society/2016/nov/19/autism-diagnosis-late-in-life-asperger-syndrome-john-harris

> talking to a friend or family. Somehow you don't feel guilty about being a burden to them, and it's just such a relief to pour it all out.
>
> However bad it gets, I seem to have an inherent desire to stay alive and, at the end of the day, it always comes back to the kids. I just couldn't do it to them.>>
>
> Mack

Another dark period in Mack's life was triggered by the terrorist attacks on the world trade centre in New York in 2001. His fledgling business was less than a year old, but things were looking good – he'd signed up some great clients for a variety of projects and by September his entrepreneurial efforts were starting to pay off.

And then those planes hit the towers. The financial world held its breath and ground to an indefinite halt as the economic fallout rippled through global financial markets. All of the projects on the books were cancelled as companies ceased outsourcing and braced themselves for uncertain times ahead. Days turned to weeks, weeks turned to months…

Because Mack had left his marriage with little but the clothes on his back and some household debt, he had no further resources left to invest in the business. And soon, he was facing the prospect of folding and taking a job – any job – in, say, London, the States, or the Far East which would mean moving away and hardly ever seeing his kids; or going bankrupt.

Those were unspeakable times that Mack still can't recollect without a wave of nausea. It took a good year or more for the business to start pulling money in again – using a completely different, less profitable but more recession-resistant model – and it was many years before he could face baked beans again. Somehow he managed to get through that experience too, albeit on his hands and knees.

16 January

During my investigations, I came across an Autie-written blog which said research had found that Auties struggle to recognise their own happiness, and that they're unable to estimate what will and won't make them happy.

I have to admit that reading this was something of a relief to me. Mack has often said things like, "I don't know what it means to be happy" or "I can't remember ever being happy". When he said stuff like that it made me feel as bad for me as for him, but now that I understand more about Auties and their black and catastrophising side, I'm able to put it in perspective a little.

So *now* when he says something like that, I remind myself of things like his ability to laugh. I don't mean when he's got a social mask on – I mean when he finds something ridiculously funny. Sometimes, when he's watching TV and I have my head in a book or am busy working in a different room, I hear a burst of uproarious, deep and infectious belly laughter – real rack-your-whole-body laughter. I've never laughed like that in my whole life and I sometimes feel a bit envious. OK, it's a fleeting moment and it doesn't mean he's 'happy', but it's perspective.

And while I know pride isn't the same as happiness, I know he's hugely proud of his kids and their achievements – you must draw a lot of pleasure from that.

He's also told me about things that have made him happy in the past. For example, he talked about his days performing music and the "extreme elation" you feel at having done something so well that people applaud you. He described a feeling of "true acceptance." We need to look back at his life and draw out more things that created these positive feelings in him. And then weave those things back into his life now.

Hey, wait a minute – rewind! I'd asked him about things that had made him *happy* in the past, but he told me instead about something that made him feel *elated*. Are we even talking about the same thing? If Mack's definition of happy is elated, then it's not surprising that he wouldn't feel that very often! Surely elation is something you'd only feel occasionally?

When *I* talk about happy/unhappy, I think in terms of a scale like: delighted – happy – pleased – content – sad – unhappy – downright miserable. But I'm beginning to suspect Mack's scale starts way higher and ends way lower. Maybe something like: ecstatic – jubilant – pleased – indifferent – sad – miserable – suicidal.

I know that, for Mack, life is all about extreme highs – such as the way he used to feel after a concert – and extreme lows – such as after dropping off his kids after an access weekend. Going forward, given the effort and energy associated with highs and the crash of exhaustion that follows when an adrenalin rush is over, I think we simply need to find ways to manage his day-to-day life better. If we make sure he's well rested and prepared for any highs, with plenty of recovery time afterwards so the lows don't have the same destructive or depressive effect, maybe we can find an equilibrium.

17 January

The article I mentioned when talking about interoception[13] claimed there's growing evidence that signals sent from our internal organs to the brain play a major role in regulating emotions and fending off both anxiety *and* depression.

If this is the case...

😕 **Key to improving mental wellbeing in autistic people who are depressed may be improving their interoception.**

Takeaways for Mack
- Do the 'mindfulness' thing from time to time, concentrating on trying to read the body's signals.
- Look back at things he used to enjoy and try to weave them back into his life now.

Takeaways for me
- Whenever he's down, encourage Mack to meditate and do exercises to improve his ability to read his body signals.
- Be aware that his habit of masking means his depression will often remain hidden.

When people are trying to help you keep calm, they often tell you to think of a happy place. The trouble is, Mack says he doesn't have one. Refusing to believe it, I've interrogated him ruthlessly in an attempt to come up with something that might help in that situation.

---

[13] The Guardian (2021), Interoception: the hidden sense that shapes wellbeing. Accessed December 2022 at:
https://www.theguardian.com/science/2021/aug/15/the-hidden-sense-shaping-your-wellbeing-interoception

I started by reminding him of the elation he used to feel during the applause that followed a concert performance. He begrudgingly conceded that, so I then suggested a few other things he's spoken fondly of in the past – golfing at his favourite course, road cycle racing, walking and playing with his dog Charlie. But although he agreed they'd all been happy places at the time, they're tinged with sadness now because he associates the memories with loss (the loss of his father who he used to golf with, the loss of his friend he used to race with, the loss of his dog…).

I tried a few other things, but they each had a negative connotation too. How about a particular piece of music? Thankfully, I had a bit more luck with that one – he credits Bryan Adams' *Summer of '69* with having saved his life before. However, unless you actually play the tune, it doesn't really help as a happy place. Why not? Ah, finally we find the rub – Mack tells me he has no imagination. He can't simply transport himself to another place, or even play a song in his head; his mind just doesn't work that way.

Turns out the inability to form a mental image of something you can't see right in front of you is called aphantasia, and it seems to be more prevalent in the autistic population. Having aphantasia means you just can't hold an image in your mind's eye. I have to admit, this surprised me. Mack has always claimed to be good at – for example – envisaging what a room might look like painted a certain colour, while I had to invest in several tester pots and still couldn't see it. Hoist on your own petard Mack! – I bet it was just your impatience and determination to get on with it that made you insist honeybee was the way to go!

And so we're going to need our own interpretation of happy place. If Mack can't use his mind to do this, it makes sense to try using his senses instead. For example, he could keep an up-to-date photo of his kids and grandpuppies in his wallet (he already has many on his phone). He could add his happy song(s) to his phone. And he could carry his favourite sandalwood scent with him in some form or other in his sensory emergency kit.

We've also talked about making plans for the future – so that he can give himself some things to look forward to when he feels well enough again.

Trauma

18 January

According to the National Autistic Society, the types of experiences Auties are prone to – such as bullying, social isolation and not being accepted by their peers – can lead or contribute to symptoms of post-traumatic stress disorder (PTSD).

PTSD is something that can affect anyone. It can develop after a single traumatic event – one that's distressing or stressful – or by repeated trauma such as abuse.

Back on page one, I mentioned that Mack was being assessed for depression and trauma as well as autism. He has since been diagnosed with PTSD. This didn't come as a huge surprise to me knowing his backstory, and more so after having watched BBC war correspondent Fergal Keane's 2022 documentary *Living with PTSD*.[14]

While the root causes of Mack's trauma are quite different from Fergal's, their symptoms are very similar.

☻ PTSD symptoms include nightmares, flashbacks, intrusive memories, distressing reminders, anxiety/fear, isolating/shutting people out, edginess/jitteriness, cold sweats/shivering inside and avoidance.

Fergal's account of what it's like to live with PTSD was a revelation to me, as much of what he was saying seemed to be describing Mack. So much so, that by the end of the

---

[14] BBC iPlayer (2022), Fergal Keane: Living with PTSD. Accessed January 2023 at:
https://www.bbc.co.uk/programmes/m0017795

programme I was pretty sure Mack was suffering from PTSD too.

Even now, 50 years on, Mack has vivid nightmares about some of the experiences of his childhood. Not *just* about that, to be fair. Last week he woke me by calling out in his sleep because he was being eaten by a wardrobe. And I'm pretty sure that never happened.

But he also suffers with the flashbacks, intrusive memories and distressing reminders that result in jitters, cold sweats, shivers and anxiety. Often, it can be something on TV that serves as a trigger – a news item, a drama, a documentary. If I spot it in time, I can quickly flick the channel. But if the trigger is a person, a behaviour or even a conversation that's taking place when we're out and about, that's not so easy to deal with.

😯 **Research indicates that autistic people may be more likely to experience traumatic life events, particularly interpersonal traumas such as bullying and physical and sexual abuse.**[15]

That said, there seems to be a lot of confusion around PTSD in the autistic population and, according to the National Autistic Society, it's hard to know for sure what the statistics are.

One of the upsides of Mack having finally hit his stone wall is that he's now been offered support – not just from Number 6 in relation to his autism diagnosis, but from psychiatric nurse Nicol for his PTSD too.

---

[15] National Autistic Society (2022), Post-traumatic stress disorder in autistic people. Accessed January 2022 at: **https://www.autism.org.uk/advice-and-guidance/professional-practice/ptsd-autism**

PTSD can be successfully treated and, with the right support, most people make a full recovery.

😶 **Mack feels he has too much on his plate to be able to deal with this right now, so this is something for later.**

Takeaways for Mack
- He doesn't need to suffer in silence – there's help out there waiting.

Takeaways for me
- Ditto. And I guess it's kept for 50 years already... It's so good to know he'll be getting support from someone who will be fully equipped to help him – when he's ready.

Gastro issues

20 January

Compared to the general population, Auties are more likely to experience digestive and gastrointestinal issues.

One obvious reason for this is sensory sensitivity – if you can't bear the texture or taste of certain things, you won't eat them, and that could limit your diet to the detriment of your health. But that's not the explanation for Mack – we could all live without sweet potato, banana and kiwi fruit.

While there have always been some foods Mack wouldn't eat, over the years he began to suffer more and more from heartburn brought on by things he'd never had problems with before. We'd try to identify the foodstuffs responsible, but he'd be fine with whatever it was one day – garlic, tomato, pepper – and not the next. So we resorted to intolerance tests, certain they'd provide the answers. They didn't though. In fact, we were left mystified when the results stated he was intolerant to, say, broccoli when he was usually fine with it, but should be OK with cauliflower when we knew he wasn't.

According to the NHS[16], lots of people get heartburn occasionally and there's often no obvious reason why. So at least he's not alone! Of the possible causes they mention, we were able to exclude a few – he's not pregnant, overweight or a smoker for example. This leaves us with

---

[16] NHS (2022), 5 lifestyle tips for a healthy tummy. Accessed January 2023 at:
https://www.nhs.uk/live-well/eat-well/digestive-health/five-lifestyle-tips-for-a-healthy-tummy/#:~:text=In%20some%20people%2C%20stress%20slows,ulcers%20and%20irritable%20bowel%20syndrome.

"certain food and drink" – such as coffee, tomatoes, alcohol, chocolate and fatty or spicy foods – or stress and anxiety.

For a few years now, Mack has taken only decaffeinated tea and coffee and only the occasional small glass of red wine. He doesn't touch spicy food of *any* kind, despite longing for a curry, as that has severe repercussions. And we both tend to shun fatty foods generally. But still the heartburn persists.

So my theory is it's mostly to do with stress. I've only once faced any prolonged anxiety in my life and that was because of a stressful situation at work. I managed a tiny bit of breakfast in the morning, but lunch was an issue – the dread of the day seemed to have blocked my swallow reflex and the most I could manage was a little soup. My head told me to eat but my insides really didn't want to – I was just too tense. While my system processed the food I *did* manage to eat without any problem, the stress only lasted a few weeks; I imagine if you were under stress day in day out for a lifetime, your system might not cope so well.

>> <<I thought I'd make Shonagh's birthday as stress-free as humanly possible so that we could all enjoy it – just a small gathering of close family. I ordered nibbles, sandwiches, canapés and cakes from a local bakery-café, and some disposable plates from Amazon so there wouldn't even be any dishwashing to do afterwards. What could be simpler?

It wasn't till we were ready to eat that I realised I'd been so focused on ordering food to accommodate other people's food fads (non-dairy, non-rice) that I'd completely forgotten about my own. £150 and not a single thing I could safely eat other than a carrot!>>

Mack

😯 **Anxiety and worry can upset the delicate balance of digestion in anyone; autistic people are more likely to have chronic problems because of chronic anxiety or stress.**

According to the NHS, "In some people, stress slows down digestion, causing bloating, pain and constipation, while in others it speeds it up, causing diarrhoea and frequent trips to the loo. Some people lose their appetite completely. Stress can also worsen digestive conditions like stomach ulcers and irritable bowel syndrome."

While it helps to follow heartburn advice – such as eating smaller, more frequent meals, avoiding triggering foods and not eating before bedtime – Mack also suffers from tummy pain and bloating occasionally after eating certain foods. Foods that the tests say he shouldn't be intolerant to. Whenever that happens, the offending item is removed from the menu, at least until such time as we've both forgotten its transgression.

And at least Mack can console himself that he doesn't react as badly, generally, as his daughter Halle does. We first noticed her food issues when she and husband Connor were staying with us during the first Covid lockdown in 2020. Within a few mouthfuls of whatever we were eating one night, her tummy ballooned to quite literally the size you'd be if you were seven months pregnant. And it was *rock* hard. Quite some party trick, but horribly uncomfortable. Intolerance tests (which her dad insisted she have done!) revealed issues with dairy and with rice, which must make food shopping and menu planning even harder in their house than in ours!

😐 **Managing stress and anxiety better should lead to an easing of any gastro issues.**

Takeaways for Mack
- Reduce general stress levels using the whole bag of Autie tricks – including interoception exercises.
- As well as sticking to decaf tea and coffee, removing carbonated drinks with caffeine can make a huge difference.
- Beware of artificial sweetener additives as these can make things worse as well.

Takeaways for me
- Take note of the foods that have this effect and don't let them over the door. This may involve a strip-search if the list includes Cadbury's crème eggs.

>> <<My body often tells me I need sugar and so I'm forever snacking on sweets or biscuits or chocolate bars. Initially, I was worried I may be diabetic but tests told me that's not the case. Still, it doesn't sound like a healthy diet, so sometimes I try to cut out the rubbish. And then I'll feel unwell or simply fall over!

> While learning about autism, I discovered that the neuro-diverse brain requires more glucose because of the higher level of processing it needs to do. Have you ever heard of a better excuse to snack?! Sadly, I'm told gummy bears should suffice. But it's one huge upside of my autism – I seem to be able to eat greater

quantities of sugary rubbish without putting on weight!>>

Mack

To limit the strain on Mack's digestive system, we try to keep our diet as simple as possible – it's pretty much all homemade because he reacts so poorly to ready-made meals. No spices, no peppers, no onions – no stock cubes even. After a typical Mack-friendly meal, I'll sneak off to some handy hideaway and scoff a chocolate treat to make up for enduring the taste tedium. Don't tell!

And we've invested in a heartburn bed wedge. The jury's still out on whether it works or not – fingers crossed though…

Medical anxiety

23 January

Whitecoat syndrome isn't specifically an Autie thing – a huge number of ordinary folk experience this. Your blood pressure is fine, but the moment a doctor or nurse tries to take it, it seems to shoot up. Or you made a doctor's appointment because you felt awful, but the moment you get to the practice your symptoms seem to have disappeared.

My Autie has been experiencing this too over the last couple of years. A lot of it is to do with the environment and the unexpected on top of any worry he might have over the underlying condition he's consulting the medics about. And which we'd all share. To date, he's got through his appointments OK thanks to the wonderful people who are our NHS. Except for the MRI.

Anyone who's a little claustrophobic struggles with an MRI, and Mack was aware he might find it difficult. To prepare for it, he did a lot of googling. So he knew what the machine looked like, how it worked, what it sounded like, how long it would take… He thought he was well prepared.

But then, without warning, they tried to strap him down – and he absolutely wasn't prepared for that! I can only imagine his reaction. They kindly called it "a dignified meltdown" and were very supportive and patient. Mack was desperate to have the MRI done as he wanted to proceed to the next stage of the process and get the treatment he needed. So he tried three times to get into that machine. And although he got a little bit further each time, they had to keep aborting. He was just way too rattled.

In the end, they rescheduled the appointment. He managed to get through the next one without any problems – he knew exactly what to expect this time – and indeed once he got in there, he found listening to the "musical patterns" of noise from the magnets calming.

😟 **The unknown and unfamiliar exacerbate any anxiety an autistic person might typically feel about medical appointments and procedures**.

> <<I've always hated needles – no idea where that came from but I don't think it's unusual. And to be honest, I don't recall having had any more anxiety about medical appointments in the past than, say, doing a business pitch or attending a business event. But I certainly find them hard now. >>
>
> Mack

Our NHS is under so much pressure these days that I'm sure they don't have time for 'difficult' patients. Imagine, you've had a long, gruelling day and then someone's being a pain about getting into the MRI machine – it would be hard to stifle your inclination to sigh!

Luckily, the NHS is staffed by kind and understanding people, and they'd likely spot the difference between someone with an anxiety and someone who's being difficult for the sake of it. But we're already finding that the mere mention of autism is enough for them to be suggesting and offering accommodations to make appointments and treatments easier.

🙂 **Having the autism diagnosis on Mack's medical file is a huge relief and is already making a difference.**

Takeaways for Mack
- Research what to expect in advance of an appointment or treatment.
- Explain to the medics that he's autistic; that familiarity with procedures helps as does counting down to difficult moments.

Takeaways for me
- Do the research with him – two heads are better than one!

> <<Till recently, I've kept fairly good health so haven't really had any medical anxiety stories to tell, unless you count the dentist. I've had a fear of dentists since childhood, following a couple of horrible incidents, and was lucky enough to eventually get onto a special desensitisation programme a few years ago.
>
> At the beginning, I wouldn't even sit in the chair. The problem wasn't necessarily getting treatment done, it was getting into the room and onto the chair in the first place and having that first injection. My dental counsellor, Rhea, tackled this by allowing me to simply sit in the room initially. Then, over a number of weeks, to lie in the chair until it no longer presented a threat. A chair that faces the door makes a huge difference – you feel much less trapped when you can see an escape route!
>
> Over two or three weeks, Rhea gently introduced Mr Whizzy the drill, Mr Pricky the needle and Mr Sucky the aspirator. The silliness kept these sessions light-hearted,

which I think contributed to reducing my anxiety; it was great to be able to laugh about it.

She handed me Mr Whizzy and let me play with it, turning it on and off so it made the noises, to see that in itself there was nothing to fear. Mr Sucky wasn't a problem until it tried to eat my tongue and I had to be rescued – doing-it-yourself dentistry is clearly not an option for me!

Mr Pricky was the biggest issue. We found that part of the problem with the injections was the type of anaesthetic they were using. It had adrenalin in it – as if I didn't have enough of that already! As a consequence of this discovery, the dentist now uses non-adrenalin stuff which doesn't escalate my heart rate nor fight with propranolol. They also showed me how thin the needles are and how flexible – in reality you hardly feel it. They numb the gum with gel and preheat the anaesthetic slightly before injecting.

When everything was put together, along with dentist Holly and dental nurse Jayne's superb handling of a nervous patient, I was finally able to receive a full programme of treatment to get back to good dental health.

One downside of non-adrenalin injections is it reduces the time they have available to work with you and increases the risk of bleeding slightly. However, I've since had some very intrusive work done – including bone removal, extractions, and removal of

>embedded roots – all without incident. A huge step forward for me, and all thanks to this approach of desensitisation.>>

Mack

24 January

Unfortunately, Mack's medical anxieties aren't limited to appointments and treatments. There's a whole layer of anxiety around any pain, sickness or unusual physical sensation way before you get to that point.

Today, there's what looks like – and I think feels like – a bruise on his leg. However, it wasn't there yesterday and he has no recollection of hurting himself, and so he's straight onto Google to explore other possibilities, including DVT. As others in his immediate family have suffered from DVT, it's not unreasonable to at least check it out and hopefully *rule* it out. Which I think he's done now, but not before he'd got himself into a tizz and had to take a herbal calm-me-down remedy (valerian) to get his heart rate/blood pressure back down. Follow that with a little distraction therapy and he'll be just fine in a while.

The tensing up of muscles caused by anxiety can lead to pain and stiffness in almost any area of the body, including the neck, shoulders, back, stomach and chest.

Did I mention we have a virtual pharmacy of just-in-case stuff in the bathroom cabinets? And first aid kits at home and in the car? And a trauma kit. And a defibrillator…

Plus we have an array of monitors to measure all sorts of things such as blood pressure, heart rate and oxygen levels. The doctor wasn't overly happy to receive a batch of readouts following a scary reaction to some meds a while back – he thought Mack had been exacerbating the problem by winding himself skyward. But Mack argues the opposite is the case.

> <<You know perfectly well when your heart's racing too fast – that's a body signal even *I* can read. When I feel a reaction like this, I try all sorts of tricks to prevent panic escalating. Counting slowly, breathing deeply, pacing calmly.
>
> Taking heart rate and blood pressure readings is just another way of me trying to take control – *willing* the readings downwards. It's hugely reassuring to watch them gradually go down. And if they don't, I know I need a little help – in this case, a little propranolol worked (an approach supported by the doctor).>>
>
> Mack

It seems strange to me that one of the ways Mack 'wills' his heart rate and blood pressure back to normal levels is to pace around. Surely it makes more sense to sit or lie down? Nope. He's too aware of his heart rate if he sits quietly, and that winds him up further. So he counts and/or breathes and paces back and forth, sitting down every now and then only for long enough to settle before taking another reading.

> <<Right now, I can hear my heart beating, my tinnitus ringing and my tummy grumbling all over the noise of the clock ticking, the boiler running and the weather outside. The last thing you want is to hear is your heartbeat getting faster and louder, so you don't want to just sit there, waiting and listening. Much better to be proactive than passive.>>
>
> Mack

The whole discussion of medical anxiety leads me perfectly into talking about catastrophising. But before I do, I just want to flag a huge upside to Mack's continual monitoring of his health. In at least one instance, it has (hopefully!) saved his life.

Mack was aware that his father had prostate issues – probably BPH – and that his uncle had prostate cancer. It didn't kill either of them and they both lived into their nineties, but it meant that Mack always had this worry at the back of his mind. And when he was diagnosed with prostate cancer, aged merely 63, he was devastated. But he only discovered this because he'd been monitoring his PSA levels privately and noticed them going up, which meant his cancer was caught relatively early.

So I for one am very glad he's proactive about his health – we'd be in a good deal more trouble right now if he had my it'll-never-happen-to-me mindset!

Catastrophising

27 January

To describe Mack as a worrier would be an understatement. His default setting is to expect the worst-case scenario and mitigate against it if possible, prepare for it if not.

I thought my tyres were fine – they got through the MOT after all – but no, they had to be replaced or I'd crash and die. He needs to have a general anaesthetic for his cancer op, so his will has to be updated. We misplaced a front door key, so all the locks had to be changed because if the key had been nicked, we'd be due a break-in.

Turns out it's not just a personality trait – it's the way Auties are wired. Hard wired.

> <<It's good to be prepared for the worst. If something happens and it's better than I expect, then it's a nice surprise. Or relief. Plus, it means I'm a natural at business continuity planning!>>
>
> Mack

Catastrophic thinking is only a problem if it spirals into something that's overwhelming, further fuelling any anxiety or depression, and reaches a point where you virtually can't function because of it. If you're hard wired to catastrophise, you can't simply stop doing it, but there are things you can do to manage it. And that's what Mack's planning and mitigating are all about.

😲 **The planning and mitigating that come with this catastrophising mindset are all about taking control, which reduces anxiety**.

And this explains Mack's control-freakery perfectly!

He's talked about the need to be in control a few times already in different contexts. For example, when he was too ill to return to work full-time after his first bout of shingles, he rearranged responsibilities in a way that allowed him to remain in overall control while working remotely. And when his heart rate/blood pressure hits the roof, he uses his monitors to will the readings back down between the pacing, counting and breathing exercises, rather than passively sitting it out. It gives his mind something to focus on rather than simply fearing the worst.

Another useful tip Mack was given by Number 6 is to look for ways of finding a positive in a negative, or even turning it around altogether. For example, a bus journey with the noisy masses might be something to be dreaded for an Autie, but download some great new music to listen to or a new book to read for the journey – suddenly there's something to look forward to about it.

☹ **Yeah, that's never going to work for Mack (he won't do buses!), but you get the idea.**

> <<Yes, I do have to be in control – there's nothing worse than *not* feeling in control – that's at least partly why I found having dental treatment so difficult. I'll gloss over my childhood experiences of alcoholic and experimental dentists; suffice to say they'd make anyone a bit wary of further dental treatment.
>
> That aside, you have to lie down on a chair – a very vulnerable position to be in – with a masked person towering over you, surrounded by all manner of scary, medieval-

looking instruments of torture. And that's before they get the needles out and the grinding begins.

I had to have a couple of extractions and was given the option of having them done under general anaesthetic [GA]. However, I know I don't react well to medication and worry that I may never come round from a GA (yes, I know I'm catastrophising!). So if there's an option, I'd rather not do that. But the moment I get into that chair my heart rate goes up, and we were concerned that with only an ordinary anaesthetic I could still have a panic attack and do a runner mid-extraction. That would be like something out of a horror movie.

So we talked about conscious sedation. I tried. Really I did. But I simply couldn't relinquish control enough to let them fix that mask to me.

We finally found a way to get through it. A very small amount of diazepam in advance of the appointment to keep me calm and get me in there, plus a tiny bit of propranolol for my heart rate/blood pressure. (All properly prescribed, of course.) This not only kept me steady enough to face the fear, but allowed me to stay with that feeling of being in control. Plus, I avoided the catastrophe of not coming round after a GA which, admit it, could happen to anyone!>>

Mack

28 January

Mack was single-handedly responsible for the loo roll shortage during the first Covid lockdown, because to have run out would have been a calamity. On the upside, we didn't have to buy more for months.

For staying in our weekend bolthole, he bought a small generator because he'd been warned there may be power outages or lightning strikes out in the sticks. Of course, it's still in its box. But you never know, some day it might come in handy.

In line with best business continuity practice, we also have spare laptops, several means of back-up and a mobile modem at home so that we can carry on working no matter what. To be fair, that's helped me out of a hole once or twice – our broadband provider isn't exactly reliable.

Takeaways for Mack
- Look for ways to turn a worry around or find something positive in it to reduce the anxiety.
- Having a plan to mitigate against a catastrophe is OK if it helps get the worry in perspective.

Takeaways for me
- Resist the temptation to roll the eyes!
- On the bright side, if he does all this worrying, *I* don't need to.
- If something's wrong, perhaps I should try to fix it before I tell him about it. But then again, he's so much better at fixing stuff!

> <<A choice few of my real-life catastrophes:
>
> I was shot at close range on the head as a kid when in the cadets. My helmet saved my life but I've had tinnitus ever since.

I fell off a ladder onto a main road when painting windows, and narrowly missed being run over by the local bus. It hurt – quite a lot – but at least I bounced in those days.

My dinghy capsized and I got entangled in the rigging and trapped underneath. Luckily the rescue boat made it to me in time.

An electric heater in my bedroom burst into flames, setting the carpet alight.

Someone jumped off the high-dive and landed on top of me, knocking me out. Fortunately, the lifeguard spotted me lying on the bottom of the pool and hauled me back out.

A plane I was on had an explosive device on it which was removed and detonated by the bomb squad. While we all lived to tell the tale, it was a pretty scary event.

I fell off a ladder fixing a skylight and landed on by back over the side of the bath. I broke three ribs but thankfully not my back.

So, bad stuff *does* happen!>>

Mack

Stimming

1 February

I'd never heard this term before, but stimming is what they call it when an autistic person makes repetitive or unusual movements or noises. Rocking is a good example, and it's something that seems to help some people manage emotions and cope with overwhelming situations.

At first, I guess we both thought, nope, Mack doesn't do that. But actually, having reflected a little more, there are a few things he does that probably qualify as stimming.

In particular, the leg shoogle (aka shake or quiver). You generally don't notice this, because his leg will be hidden under a table when this is happening. On a bad day, both legs can go off together and if you're sitting on a bench beside him, it's like being on top of the washing machine on its spin cycle!

When he's not sitting down, he might instead be twiddling something – anything – in his hand, over and over. He's not usually aware he's doing it. Pacing is also listed as an example of stimming, and Mack does this when he's anxious or feeling caged in.

I confess, I surreptitiously googled 'Is it only autistic people who stim?', because although it hasn't happened in a long time, there's a thing I do when I'm extremely anxious or distressed. My angst manifests itself as a pain in my right hand, so I splay it wide and then clench it tight, splay, clench, splay, clench… and this seems to alleviate the pain.

Hits seem to suggest that while it's most common in people on the spectrum, pretty much everyone stims now and again. Examples include foot tapping, nail biting, cracking your knuckles, twirling your hair or drumming your fingers.

😮 **This is generally a response to anxiety or sensory overload. Stimming can reduce sensory input because focusing on one action can reduce the impact of an overwhelming environment. It's a way of keeping calm.**

<<A client gave me this little cornelian stone many years ago – it's shiny now that I've played with it so much by turning it over and over and over in my pocket – I wonder if he suspected I was autistic?!>>

Mack

😕 **Nothing to worry about then…**

Takeaways for Mack
- If it's having the effect of keeping him calm, or of calming him down before or after something that makes him anxious, it's a good thing.
- Try a variety of different fiddling objects/stim toys to find what works best.

Takeaways for me
- Remember to tighten the screws on that bench – I'm convinced they're coming loose!
- Instead of pinning his knee still, check in case there's something preying on him that I'm not aware of, and suggest something that might help him chill out a bit.

Repetitive behaviour

2 February

This is a tricky one as I'm not exactly sure what qualifies as repetitive behaviour. Some sources seem to use the term interchangeably with stimming, others suggest stimming is merely a type of repetitive behaviour. I think a wider definition makes more sense, as Mack does a lot of things time and time again that couldn't possibly qualify as 'a way of keeping calm'.

It would be great if repetitive behaviour could be something like, say, doing housework on a Monday, shopping on a Tuesday, washing on a Wednesday… because it would take the pain out of chores if they could be as automatic as brushing your teeth in the morning. But we don't really have any kind of timetable for anything in our household. And would this not be a habit rather than a behaviour?

During the diagnosis stage, I was asked about Mack's 'peculiarities' – anything odd or different about his behaviours to most people's. One of the things that sprang to mind was that in the 22 years I'd known him, he'd gone through 29 cars (yes, I painstakingly recalled and counted every one of them). That's got to be unusual. But is it repetitive behaviour?

I guess, for a clever guy, he can be remarkably daft in some ways – as in lacking common sense – which could maybe be put down to repetitive behaviour. For example, he'll have a fruit scone for supper and then have heartburn all night. Most of us would immediately resolve to never do that again, or at least not for supper. But not Mack. He'll make that same resolution but then he'll do it again, and again and again – although to be fair these instances may be spread over weeks and months. Is *that* repetitive behaviour? (If it is, I could come up with *hundreds* of examples!) Or is it just some kind of memory problem?

Then there are plugs and locks. Everything must be switched off at night – and certain things unplugged too – and every door and window needs to be checked and rechecked. (Long gone are my single days when I could happily scoot off to work with nothing but the yale on the front door and leaving the bedroom window open.) It's like Fort Knox for us now, wherever we are. I'm not sure if *this* is repetitive behaviour or just that he's a bit of a safety/security nut.

>> <<As a child, I had a big issue with electrical sockets – switches couldn't be in any position other than off when not being used. I'd then go round the room sometimes up to a dozen times, counting to 10 to make sure the switch didn't go back on by itself. Maybe this was a bit of OCD [obsessive-compulsive disorder]. Or it could have been the result of a fire in my bedroom caused by an electrical appliance blowing out. Regardless, I did this socket checking and rechecking routine for years. Thankfully, it's well under control now!>>

Mack

During my investigations, I found that the leg shoogle I mentioned earlier – his stimming – definitely qualifies as repetitive behaviour. The calming kind.

But routine also comes up frequently under this topic. For many Auties, routine is very important because it reduces the anxiety that comes with the unexpected. So everything they do may need to be done in the same way each time, and even the activities they do each day may need to be done in the same order. Mack certainly used to run his professional life along these lines.

> <<I found that following a routine definitely helped with the more stressful aspects of work. For example, I'd approach business meetings the same way each time. I would always be early and well prepared. I would then start the meeting with the usual pleasantries and the obligatory teas and coffees, giving myself time to settle into the meeting which was important. For meetings where I was in control of the venue, I could choose my seating position – always with a clear 'escape' route in sight and my back to the light – so that I felt most at ease.
>
> As is the nature of compliance work however, some meetings were adversarial. If my adversary were in charge of the venue, they would control the seating arrangements to their own advantage, steering me to a position that would leave me uncomfortable and anxious. As all the best interrogators do! When that happened, I would simply look to turn the tables on them by pacing the room and standing from time to time with my back to the window. This forced them to look up at me and keep turning their heads. Not only did this give me back a measure of control, but I found the pacing itself calming.
>
> If challenged about this behaviour, I would simply cite sciatica or similar.>>
>
> Mack

3 February

In his personal life, I struggle to think of any routines Mack has other than:

- Conducting his security checks every night.
- Visiting the loo whenever he leaves home whether he needs or not. Unless that's simply a prostate thing!
- Arriving very early for, well, anything and everything really.

I'd love him to have a few more routines, especially around the house. For example, it would be great if he could put things back in the *right* place rather than the nearest. That would give me a fighting chance of being able to find them again. However, I know for sure he'd say that if I hadn't left these things lying around in the first place, he wouldn't have had to put them away. Which is fair enough. Mack is much tidier than me, but don't go looking in his cupboards – I guarantee that everything will burst out and smack you on the head.

It's a pain in the neck when he tidies up while I'm in the middle of something though – which he does frequently! Today, for example, I'd pushed the heavy and moveable furniture into the middle of the room. My plan was to dust the skirtings and hoover into the corners, then dust the hard furniture and hoover the soft furniture then, finally, put everything back so that I could hoover the middle of the room. Sounds like a great plan, doesn't it? Not when you've got a Mack, helpfully putting everything back behind you before you've even *started* hoovering! But I admit it's lovely of him to try to help…

It's much the same when I try to cook something. I start by looking out all the ingredients and all the utensils I need, then I do any prep required and start the cooking – often following a recipe because I'm a bit rubbish behind a pinny at the best of times. I'll be halfway through and then wonder if I'm going mad. I'm sure I'd looked out the olive oil, the garlic, the grater and so on. But the foodstuffs have all been returned to the cupboard already and the utensils are now in the dishwasher – it's not just that I haven't *finished* with them yet, I've often not even *started*! [Sighs.] Unless of course that's the idea. I have to admit there have been a considerable number of my cooking attempts/experiments over the years that even the kids agreed were better off in the bin than on their plates!

While Mack definitely needs to plan and prepare for things, he doesn't seem to need much in the way of an obvious or formal structure. He's always been less organised (outside of work) and more spontaneous than me.

I have a similar dislike of plans changing with little warning, but it's not because it creates anxiety for me. Usually, it's because I've created a different expectation in my mind of how to spend the day and will be disappointed not to be able to get on with whatever my plan had been.

Mack has become known over the years among friends and family for cancelling. To the point where we've probably thought of that trait in terms of repetitive behaviour – a layman's definition, that is, not the stimming/structure/routine definition my investigations have largely been coming up with. However, the reason for this has become abundantly clear to us since the autism diagnosis. Mack has never before managed how much may be on his plate at any one time; he's always just said 'yes' to anything and everything and then found himself overloaded or overwhelmed. That's when he steps on the brakes and cancels.

By following Autie advice to space events out, allowing enough psych-up and recuperation time for each, we can hopefully quash this habit.

Several of the tricks Mack has used to reduce medical anxiety can also be used to reduce general or social anxiety, making it less likely that he'll want to cancel arrangements. For example, scoping out a venue beforehand – in real life or online – and getting an advance copy of an agenda, programme, procedure or even menu depending on what the occasion is. These things all help to create an expectation of what will happen so there are fewer surprises to deal with on top of the sensory burden.

😮 **Repetitive behaviour in the context of autism means stimming and routines, which can be helpful in keeping calm and mitigating against anxiety and the unexpected.**

I think we need to look at the repeating of mistakes (such as the fruit scones) under a different microscope – memory maybe. Or perhaps this is just Mack and nothing at all to do with autism…

😐 **Again, nothing to worry about now that we have an understanding of the autistic mind.**

Takeaways for Mack
- If repetitive behaviours become a problem, re-examine the cause of any increased stress or anxiety.

Takeaways for me
- If Mack keeps using his new box of tricks to stave off anxiety and overload, repetitive behaviours shouldn't become a problem.

Rules

5 February

Compliance seems an odd choice of career for someone who dislikes confrontation. Clients employ compliance consultants for advice, but it seems to me that for the most part the last thing they want to do is actually comply – they generally want advice on how to get away with not complying. And they can get very creative in their suggestions of how they might do that.

Such discussions can get very heated, so I can sympathise with Autie Donald's approach of listening to their inventive proposal, telling them "No" and simply hanging up. But if you're too polite to do that – or are interested in keeping the business – that's not really an option.

Instead, you have to quote the rules and explain the consequences of not following them. Again and again, and in as many different ways as you can. I know it would wear me down.

So why do it?

> <<Well, because it's all about rules; there's no dubiety. If you follow them you won't have any problems, if you don't you could go to jail.
>
> Clients can argue till they're blue in the face, but a rule is a rule so they can't undermine your confidence – if you know your stuff you know you're right and you're on solid ground, however aggressive they might become. It's not personal, it's the law.>>
>
> Mack

OK, I get that. But it must be stressful, especially when it's you against everyone else in the room.

Even before getting into compliance, Mack's career meanderings seem to have been rules and procedures based. Banker, legal clerk, system analyst…

This isn't to say Mack doesn't rail against rules from time to time. Tennis for example. He hates that you get a second chance to serve if you fluff your first attempt, so he'll spend Wimbledon fortnight ranting about that. And he doesn't worry over much about what goes in which bin – I'm the one who gets in a fankle over my browns and greens and blues.

In general though, Mack is a law abider and finds it hard to tolerate people who flaunt legality or the rules of convention we collectively live by. So when there's an accident or an altercation, he'll step forward if he sees things going in the wrong direction – such as the innocent party getting the blame or coming off worst. When dashcams first became a thing, he took great delight in sending footage to the police of any dangerous driving. Still does.

During the first lockdown in 2020, Mack went out for an essential food shop. Everyone was queuing outside – as only so many were allowed in at one time – and wearing face masks. One bloke, however, ignored the queue and the sanitiser station, went straight up to the counter and started abusing the shop assistant. No mask or anything. Mack saw red and "folded him up and bundled him out of the shop", earning himself a round of applause and a free basketful. He wouldn't normally react like that but a combination of anger over the rule-breaking and rudeness, and anxiety over potential super-spreading, along with the armour of the mask, numbed any anxiousness he would have been feeling.

6 February

We followed Covid rules to the nth degree right up until the last of the restrictions were lifted. This meant that when son Stuart was eventually allowed to visit, we had to sit outside huddled in blankets. Stuart had to bring his own lunch, pee at the bottom of the garden and wash his hands under the garden tap. Thankfully, he's long-suffering and forgiving by nature.

Not all the Covid rules were dictated by the government though. Halle used to be a nurse so she was very hot on infection control. This meant that I was virtually hosed down on my return from the weekly grocery shopping, and every item had to be disinfected before being stored in the fridge or cupboards. Good practice in the early days of the pandemic. But even after Halle and Connor returned to their Glasgow home after lockdown, Mack dutifully continued this practice for weeks, possibly months!

And while we're on the subject of food, let's not forget use-by and best-before dates. Officially, only use-by dates qualify as a rule, don't you think? With best-before being simply guidance. I happily ignore both and will carry on eating something until it smells or tastes really unpleasant. And in all my years, I've only poisoned myself once. (I reheated a chicken casserole one too many times – won't be doing that again!)

Mack, however, starts getting twitchy even on the named date, and definitely won't eat anything that's exceeded it even by a day. To be fair, I'm not sure this is to do with a need to follow rules though – it's just as likely to be due to his oversensitive digestive system.

When researching why rules are important to Auties, I found a lot of answers to do with predictability and the difficulties of navigating a neurotypical world.

One study I came across[17] – albeit dating back a bit – found that autistic children reported a higher level of frustration with rule-breaking than the control group. When rules were being broken, their brains showed an over-active insula – that's the area of the brain triggered by intense emotion.

😮 **Broken rules are even more distressing to autistic people than being excluded.**

Some Auties will follow rules pedantically regardless of whether or not they understand them. Others, like Mack, will think more critically about the importance and intention of a rule before deciding if and when to follow it.

Because Auties can't filter out extraneous sensory information, their brains process everything. They also experience things more intensely. When you put these two things together, it results in overload and/or a sense of chaos. Rules – and the routine of following rules – bring order to that chaos and make the world a safer, more predictable place with more consistent outcomes.

So choosing a career based around rules suddenly makes a lot of sense.

Perhaps the extent of your rule-following depends on where you are on the spectrum and on the amount of sensory input you have to handle – rules and routines reduce the amount

---

[17] Spectrum (2011) Playing by the rules. Accessed February 2023 at:
https://www.spectrumnews.org/opinion/playing-by-the-rules

of overstimulation you're exposed to because there's less to think and worry about.

> <<For me, it was never the work itself that was stressful. I enjoyed the research, the debates over interpretation, the problem-solving and presenting solutions. And I always made sure I knew my stuff and was well prepared.
>
> The stress was to do with the environment, the unknown and interactions with difficult people – innocently difficult because they didn't understand, or obstructively difficult because they didn't want to comply. I've always found confrontation nerve-wracking.
>
> People judge you on how you perform or present so, if anything, I'll be *over*-prepared for a visit. I work things out to the last detail, and control the meeting in line with the agenda to reduce interaction as much as possible. Precision is the key – it's more down to planning rather than clear thinking at the time. Even so, I'll be completely exhausted afterwards.>>
>
> Mack

Mack recalls the days when he used to lecture in the US. He'd go over there a couple of days beforehand to give himself time to recover from the journey, and then work hard preparing so that he had a clear path to follow and solid script memorised. God help anyone who deviated him from it.

Afterwards, he'd head straight for the airport and sleep soundly till he got home. To an extent, he took it in his stride because he was lecturing on a rules-based subject he knew inside out. But if someone asked him out socially during the trip? He couldn't do it.

Mack got on particularly well with the compliance officer of one of his client firms in England, Jack, and indeed would count him among his friends. In the early days of their business relationship, Jack would invite Mack to stay at his place rather than a hotel, which he did a couple of times. But he found it too much. By the time he'd done a full day's work with the requisite interviews and interactions at the client's office, he was simply too exhausted to cope with a social situation, however much he enjoyed Jack's company and hospitality.

Instead, he had to shut himself away in a hotel at the end of the day with a room service meal, and then go straight to sleep because he was so tired. He never understood why he was dogged by such fatigue. At that stage, no one knew.

😕 **It would be rare for Mack, as a critical thinker, to insist on a rule that's plain silly, so I just need to check he's not following a rule due to a default setting in his brain.**

Takeaways for Mack
- He can break any rule he wants – so long as he doesn't also break the law, obviously.

Takeaways for me
- If Mack feels the need to follow a rule/law/regulation, it's better to go along with it than subject him to the anxiety involved in breaking it.

Other differences

Memory

9 February

Under listening, I mentioned that there are often occasions when I'll come home to find Mack has made something entirely different for dinner than whatever it was we'd agreed to have. So that salmon I'd defrosted will end up in the bin, because there's no way he'll eat it the following day – it will have exceeded its eat-within time by then.

Sometimes this happens because he hasn't actually heard me. His ears have picked up my words and his tongue has sent an automated response without his brain being engaged in any way whatsoever. It's like an out-of-office reply politely set to 'yes'. Rubber-ear listening. But there are other times when the salmon will have been *his* idea. So what's going on there?

Memory is endlessly fascinating, but Mack's one confounds me.

First, there's the whole salmon thing. We'll have had that discussion at breakfast time and he's clearly forgotten it by mid-to-late afternoon, even when it's his suggestion.

Second, there are his favourite stories. If someone tells you the same story two or three times over a 20-year period, you don't think much of it. It's like a favourite film – you can enjoy the very best ones many times, though perhaps not in quick succession. But there are some stories he's told me so many times that I could recount them back to him almost word for word. Does he *really* not remember he's told me them before, or does he just enjoy the telling of them so much that he doesn't care?

Third, there's his visual memory, and that's something else altogether!

Although scientific journals say there's still no proof that there's such a thing as a photographic memory, it's defined as the ability to recall something in detail, just like a photograph. Mack can do this, and Number 6 confirm that quite a number of their Auties do too – though by no means all.

I like to make cheeky use of this gift when I've lost something by asking him if he can close his eyes and picture where it is. And if he's seen it, he can usually tell me. To be fair, this is probably at least partly explained by the sensory sensitivity thing – he visually takes in way more than the rest of us.

> <<Shonagh often asks me where she might have left something – and even through I've not touched it, I'll likely have walked past it in my usual scanning mode. She'll ask me to picture where I last saw it, and about 90% of the time I get it right. The other 10% I get a frown if I've sent her to the wrong shelf! So I've learned to caveat my answers now, suggesting places she might like to look, just in case!>>
>
> Mack

This ability doesn't stop him misplacing his own stuff though – wallet, keys, etc. And he cheats by putting these bleeper things on them so he can find them when he does lose them. After all, who wants to use their head when they can play with a gadget?!

Mack is also great at recognising people – even if he's only met or seen them once before. And even if that was aeons ago. I'm very envious of that gift because I sometimes wonder if I have the opposite problem – prosopagnosia (face blindness). I'm OK if someone has a very distinctive feature I can cling on to. A facial scar, two different-coloured eyes, a whacky hairdo. And I'm OK with people I've met several times – but it generally does take several meetings!

😲 **Due to increased activity in the visual areas of their brain, autistic people can have an almost photographic memory.**

> <<Being able to picture things in my mind has helped me in many ways throughout life.
>
> Way back in high school, we were asked as part of a Latin exam to translate a piece of text from Virgil's Aeneid. I could clearly recall both the original Latin text and the English version from when we'd covered this in class, and I recognised the start of the text as being from about two-thirds of the way through. So I quickly dumped that memory onto paper, finishing the exam 40 minutes early.
>
> While I was pleased to get full marks, there was a rather pointed comment from the teacher who'd marked it along the lines of, "It would have been good if you'd actually stopped where the text did with your translation!" Oops.>>
>
> Mack

10 February

Mack has noticed his photographic memory works better for objects and words than for numbers. But of more concern to him is that it doesn't work well when he's tired or unwell. Sometimes this would hamper him in his professional life, bringing his performance down to the level of a mere mortal.

For almost 40 years he'd been working with lots of rules and regulations across multiple laws, handbooks and documents. His memory enabled him to go straight to the right page to find whatever he needed to answer a client's question or defend a position. His head being a biological search engine!

A few years ago, after having been prescribed medication for shingles, his memory wouldn't function in this way for two or three months. He found this distressing as well as inconvenient. Fortunately, things gradually returned to normal as he recovered.

☹ Too little restful sleep can result in mood changes and anxiety, which in turn contribute to problems with memory – for anyone, not just autistic people.

Takeaways for Mack
- If his memory isn't working, it probably means he's overtired and needs to rest.
- And/or he needs a sugar or glucose boost. Or water.

Takeaways for me
- He'll be able to find more 'lost' things for me when he's firing on all cylinders – there's no point asking when he's in zombie mode or agitated about something.
- If I keep him well rested, I'll be able to continue enjoying access to this superpower!

While my online investigations suggest that Auties do at least as well as their neurotypical peers at remembering information presented visually (and often excel at it as Mack does), there's a lot of variation when it comes to verbal working memory. Much may depend on the kind of information they're trying to remember and whether on hearing it they had to process it as well as remember it.

According to Psychology Today[18], studies confirm that when remembering information, Auties don't use their long-term memory, visual strategies, or even contextual clues. Instead, they rehearse or repeat things over and over again. While this can be useful in remembering little things, it's not the best strategy. Clearly, Mack didn't repeat 'salmon' often enough to remember it by dinner time!

Does this shed any light on the repeat stories? Perhaps it does. If you don't automatically store things in your long-term memory (such as 'I've told Shonagh the one about…'), then I guess it's bound to crop up again.

A theme that came up a few times when I was reading about Auties' memories was to do with remembering behaviours. While Auties can store and recall incredible amounts of factual information about all sorts of things – particularly any special interest they might have – they'd often write themselves reminders about behaviours that didn't come naturally. 'Hug partner today', for example.

I know a lot of people are brought up in the kind of families that say 'love you' lots. That wasn't something we did in our family, so it doesn't come naturally to me. Mack's

---

[18] Psychology Today (2020), Autism and Memory. Accessed February 2023 at:
https://www.psychologytoday.com/intl/blog/keep-it-in-mind/202004/autism-and-memory

family didn't do it either, but somewhere along the line Mack must have decided it was important, so he does it a lot – which is lovely. I've still not mastered it myself and am wondering whether I, like the Auties I've read about, should keep a little notebook with reminders like that!

In one of the stories I came across, a mother asked her autistic son why he never said 'love you' back. The boy clearly remembered saying 'love you' to her when he was six years old, so was thoroughly confused by the fact that she wanted to hear it again. This tickled me, but maybe it's because I could see myself in that little boy! Despite not qualifying as an Autie, it would appear that I do share some of their typical traits and could probably do with adopting some of their wiles to get by.

Then there are the circular or never-ending debates – which I'm guessing must share an explanation with the salmon thing. For example, "Do we need to redo the crumbling floor in the outbuilding [at the bolthole], and if so, what with? Cement, slabs, decking, gravel, crushed chips…?" To my mind, the answer is, "No, why bother? I'm sure the money could be better spent elsewhere." But he doesn't like that answer so he'll persevere. He'll wear me down to the point of accepting that it's going to happen. But the remainder of the conversation is the same. "What with? Cement, slabs, decking…"

Eventually, he'll decide what he thinks is best and I'll agree, glad to hear the end of it. But it's not. The end of it I mean. A day or two later, we'll be back to, "…what with?" as though the last conversation (sorry, monologue) had never happened.

I had a colleague a bit like this once, Caitlyn. She was lovely, but she would chatter away about an issue for ages before finally deciding, "Yes, that's exactly what I'll do – thanks for your help!" I hadn't said a word.

Learning and working things out

12 February

So, Auties are great at learning – just, as we know, not necessarily by listening! There are references everywhere to their fascination with the world around them and their zest or hunger for learning. That's definitely Mack – although I'd have called it finding out rather than learning per se. But then I've only known him since we were both long past the formal and further education stages of our lives. Ask him how to do anything – anything at all – and if he doesn't know already, he'll soon find out.

And because Auties think differently, they're often creative and great at problem-solving too. Yes, that describes Mack as well. Let's gloss over the fact that he's managed to create a good few of the problems in the first place – he's supposed to be great at planning, but his enthusiasm usually sweeps him away before any plan is thought through and 'signed off'! Patience is not Mack's strongest suit. He'd rather crack on with something and if it goes wrong, well that's just a learning experience – try, try again.

An example would be the rebuilding of a 1950s classic car – a project he undertook during the year of the Covid lockdowns.

> <<The poor old wreck hadn't run for years, but the pandemic provided a great opportunity to get it going again.
>
> I had done lots of research and downloaded manuals and illustrations to help with the rebuild. But instructions of any kind are really just a fallback – I'd much rather get on with it

and refer to them only if I have to – when I get really stuck.

I'd ordered all the bits I thought we needed and my mechanic friend Mark and I set about it. After only a few days of work, we were delighted with ourselves – the only thing left to do was top up the water, oil and petrol and it should be ready to go. Everything was going swimmingly up to that point. And then we noticed there was more oil on the floor than in the car – and no obvious reason why.

So we had to take everything back to pieces again, only to discover a hairline crack along the bottom of the engine which needed specialist welding. This meant the engine had to be taken out of the car and loaded into Mark's van – a much hairier task than it sounds. It was *unbelievably* heavy! In fact, we nearly caused the van to rear up on its hind wheels as we struggled to get it far enough into the back to be stable, and it's surprising we didn't do ourselves an injury in the process. We should have used engine lifts.

And when we were dismantling everything, we really should have taken note of how to put it all back together again. But we didn't. So when we tried reassembling it two weeks later, we couldn't get it to work. It took us aeons, laboriously studying diagrams and using trial and error to finally get it running again. Which thankfully it did.

I know the moral of the story is to read the instructions first, or to do plans/notes along the way, whatever. But really, who has the patience for that?!>>

> Mack

13 February

Auties are persistent – check – good at problem-solving – definitely – and generally have good if not exceptional memories – yep. When you put it all together, you're talking about a pretty impressive skillset.

I was quite amused however, to come across "…have the ability to pursue personal theory or perspective despite conflicting evidence"[19]. It made me laugh because when Number 6 asked me about Mack's 'peculiarities' during the diagnosis process, his wild theories did spring to mind.

"I've only had this pain/problem since the vaccine." Hmm, I'm pretty sure you were complaining about that well before the vaccine.

"Computer viruses were invented by companies with a commercial interest in selling solutions." Really?

"There's no way Covid was a natural phenomenon – it was a dastardly plot… and they were *way* too quick to find a vaccine." Now you sound a bit like Donald Trump.

The difficulty with his various and often crazy ideas is that sometimes, just *sometimes*, he might be right about something – they say a stopped clock is right twice a day after all.

---

[19] Autisable (2016), Blessings of Aspergers/Autism. Accessed February 2023 at:
https://autisable.com/2016/09/03/blessings-of-aspergersautism

On a similar vein, there are his crass generalisations. So, for example, "All Audi drivers are [replace with a word of your own choosing]". Given quite a few friends and family drive Audis, that sounds like dangerous territory to me! Virtually begging for a slap on the head.

As for working things out – well, this is something that still exasperates me a little. I ask Mack to explain or show me how to do something, but he just goes ahead and does it. So I ask him how he did it, because I want to know for next time, and he just looks at me blankly.

> <<It used to infuriate me at school – I got all the answers right, in a fraction of the time it took most of the class, and yet they'd mark me right down because I hadn't put my workings. The way I saw it, it was just stupid to make you laboriously work things out on paper when the answers were already clear in your head!>>
>
> Mack

(Evidently, he's still smarting over that one!) It's a point of view, I guess, but it doesn't help *me*. I still can't get the printer to work, or my satnav to update or my phone to pair and I'd *really* like to know how... Just as well he didn't choose a career in training.

😲 The autistic brain works differently, and autistic people find it difficult to explain things they just *know*.

Do they 'just know' though? Or do they have a different way of working things out that they don't realise or simply can't (or won't!) explain?

When Mack *does* try to explain something, he seems to become a little inarticulate. "You just do this, and then that…" But this and that are so quick I miss them.

There's nothing Mack cares about more than his family, and he'll do anything and everything for us. So maybe all I need to do is press home the message that he really needs to share some of the stuff he's got locked in that preternatural brain of his. Otherwise, how are we going to manage if he has a genuine catastrophe and we're left without him? Or would that be too brutal?!

😕 **I don't see any way round having to take the rough with the smooth on this one.**

Takeaways for Mack
- Try to show people how he gets things done.
- Be more patient – we'll catch up eventually.

Takeaways for me
- Find someone else to explain or show me how to do the techy things I struggle with.

<<It's so much quicker to just *do* something than it is to explain.

The downside is you then have to do everything yourself – although at least if you do, you know it's right *and* that it's done on time. Oh, that's my 'control-freakery' talking again!

A couple of months ago, my daughter and son-in-law's car alarm kept going off, and they couldn't switch it off or start the car. The immobiliser thought the car was being broken into, despite them using the remote key. They took it to the garage who spent a day investigating, changed the battery in the key and charged £120. But the problems continued. Halle was so frustrated she wanted to sell the car – inconvenience aside, the constant racket was just too embarrassing. Now, the garage wanted £1,000 to replace the control modules and the remotes.

When the kids called me for advice, the first question I asked was about the battery. Of course, they assured me it couldn't be that because the garage had changed the battery for them.

I spent goodness knows how long googling for alternative explanations and eliminating them one by one, till I eventually picked up the phone to a dealer I was on good terms with. He kindly sent me the technical handbook so that I could again eliminate any other possibilities – quicker and easier to do that myself than have to go through it with someone else. The next time they were through with the car, still bemoaning its behaviour, I asked for the key and simply changed the battery. With one of the right thickness this time!

Working things out isn't hard – you just need to do the research if you don't already know the answer! (Which actually I did – did I not suggest it was the battery in the first place?!)>>

Mack

Researching is a whole other 'thing' of course, and it's all bound up with an Autie's need to know. And they really do *need* to know stuff!

Before I move on to that though, while we're still on the subject of working things out, I want to tell you a story about the grandpuppies, Archie and Haggis.

Mack loves them both to bits and, interestingly, given they're polar opposites in terms of personality, he relates to both of them in different ways.

Archie belongs to daughter Halle and her husband Connor. He's a King Charles spaniel, particularly cute but a wee feartie. Archie's not just scared of hoovers, but of the cardboard cores of toilet rolls, empty plastic bottles and pretty much anything unfamiliar. He's also not at all keen on wintry weather. His expression on his first-ever sight of snow spoke volumes – clear as day, he said, "I'm not going out in *that*!" And, as if he hadn't already made his feelings perfectly clear, he dug his little heels in firmly and pulled back with all his might.

Adventurer Haggis, on the other hand, couldn't get enough of the stuff – he went absolutely crazy, bounding around in it like an over-excited kangaroo. Haggis belongs to son Stuart. He's a cocker spaniel, every bit as cute as Archie but a complete tearaway and destroyer of anything remotely chewy. While Archie is happy to sit for a cuddle, Haggis can only cope with that for a moment or two before he's off again.

One day the kids decided to test how clever the dogs were. One of the tests was to place a treat on the floor, let them see you putting a blanket over it and time how long it took them to reach it.

Haggis won, but I seriously think that Archie should have. Yes, it took him longer, but that was because when he realised he was struggling to get the treat by himself, he stopped and asked for help. How smart is that?! Only when it became obvious that no one was going to help him did he get back to figuring it out for himself.

I think he should have been given bonus points for using his common sense. Note for Haggis *and* Mack (and this is the point of this little story!): a high IQ is pointless if you don't have the wit to ask for help when you need it.

Persevering and perseverating

16 February

"I've started so I'll finish." I know that's a *Mastermind* catchphrase, but it also epitomises Mack.

I can only recall one thing that Mack started but *didn't* finish. We were renovating a flat. On the very first day – an hour or so into the job perhaps – he fell off a ladder, breaking three ribs in the process. So he *couldn't* finish – and nor could I because I suddenly had a fair bit of nursing and mollycoddling to do. Luckily, we knew someone who knew someone…

Generally, the job gets done no matter what. I waste a fair bit of breath on, "Why not take a break?", "Isn't that enough for one day?" or "There's no rush – we can finish this another time." But unless I physically disable him, he won't stop. Afterwards, there's the inevitable, "I think I've overdone it..." I bite my tongue.

When I ask him *why* he needs to do a job all in one go, he says things like, "Someone's got to do it." Which isn't always true – some of these projects seem completely unnecessary to me. Pushed a little further, he admits that once he's decided that something needs to be done, it simply preys on his mind until it's finished. Whether it's a manual or mental task, it worries away at him so he finds it best just to crack on with it.

If it's to do with work – a client query, say – he'll find himself fretting about it at 4am and, knowing he won't get back to sleep while it's on his mind, he simply gets up and deals with it.

Perseverance is definitely one of his strengths. But is it an Autie thing?

I googled to find out, but all my hits were about autism and *perseveration*. I thought I'd mistyped at first, but no, perseveration seems to be a real word from the world of psychology.

😲 **Perseveration is when someone continually repeats a thought or behaviour as though they're fixated on it or stuck in a loop.**

Oh no! He's got another '*thing*'...!

After doing a bit more digging however, I've decided that this maybe isn't as scary as it sounds. It seems that we can all perseverate occasionally – for example, looking in the same place for something several times because you're sure it *must* be there. I definitely do that. Almost every day! But it's common for Auties to perseverate because of the challenges they tend to have with managing anxiety and processing information. It's often a sign of sensory overload.

My investigations suggest that there are three types of perseveration – verbal, motor and cognitive.

Verbal is where you repeat yourself a lot. Wait a minute – is that not just parenthood? OK, a better example would be where someone has a fascination that he or she feels so keenly that they have to tell you about it – the same thing about it – *all* the time. To the point where you've not only become an authority on it yourself, but it's driving you mad. Even that just sounds like your average football fan. A more depressing example is where you ask a series of unrelated questions and just get the first answer on repeat to all of them. That definitely sounds like overload but, thankfully, it's not something I've ever noticed happening to Mack.

Motor perseveration is the same thing but with movement rather than words – usually facial expressions, or hand or arm movements. I'm not sure I'd be able to tell the difference between that and stimming. Or Tourette's. But I'm not going to worry about that just now, as I've not noticed Mack doing anything like this other than the things I'd already decided, rightly or wrongly, were stimming.

Cognitive perseveration is when you can't stop thinking about something – such as going over a conversation or a worry time and time again in your mind. That doesn't sound like much of a concern if it's constructive, or even if it's a bit pointless. And we all do a bit of that, don't we? But it's not so good if it's negative, as that road can lead to dark places. Unlike stimming, which is calming, cognitive perseveration is an unconscious way of coping that can exacerbate a problem or feeling. I fear Mack scores quite highly on this one.

> <<We were putting up a potting shed. To be fair, it was a big shed and it took a while, but we're only talking wood, felt and a bunch of nails.
>
> However, it clearly got on the neighbour's goat. He came storming round and had a tantrum that would have done a two-year-old proud. I wasn't there – I'd left Shonagh tapping in the last few nails on the roof felt – but I watched it on the security camera afterwards and saw him in frenzied full flap. It didn't help that Shonagh's reaction to his behaviour was a barely stifled giggle, but I was absolutely livid!

> Even now, Shonagh thinks it's funny. She desperately wanted me to leave it alone and not exacerbate the situation but to be honest, I've never got over it. It still replays in my mind, again and again, and it sticks in my craw to even be polite to him in passing now.>>

Mack

17 February

So, does perseveration shed (ha-ha) a new light on any of Mack's behaviours that I hadn't already found a satisfactory explanation for?

Could it be why he keeps eating fruit scones at bedtime when he ought to have learned they give him heartburn? Hmm, don't think so.

Could it be why he repeats the same stories many times? Well, not the ones that are spread over a few decades – I have the distinct impression that the perseverating, or ruminating, is a short-term thing.

However, I'm sure it *does* explain why, when he gets an idea in his head, he talks round in circles about it time and time again. He's just thinking out loud. I don't think it's anything to do with sensory overload though – my money's on anxiety. The fruit scones and the repeat stories are more likely to be memory issues.

But I digressed, didn't I? I'd been googling autism and perseverance before finding my attention hijacked by perseveration. So, let's rewind a bit. Not only did I not find any particular link between perseverance and autism, but most of Mack's late diagnosis group took a different approach, at least when it came to overload-of-work issues.

I believe they were talking about how they handled workload, and Mack explained that he couldn't leave an email undealt with because it would worry away at him, no matter what it was about. Now that I have the official parlance, I should say he would *perseverate* over it! Allowing emails to build up would prevent Mack from getting a good night's sleep and make the next day harder to face. He advocates going to bed with a clean sheet, so to speak.

However, Mack tells me most of the group found that they could only handle so much. When they were inundated with emails, they could almost feel themselves shutting down, so they were more likely to take the 'chuck-it bucket' approach. Which is exactly what it sounds like – anything that's just too much is chucked, ignored or, in the case of emails, deleted!

Mack loves the idea of the chuck-it bucket, but he could no more change his spots than the proverbial leopard could its habits of a lifetime.

Oh, hold up – we have another terminology trip hazard here. Perseveration vs rumination; it appears they're not the same thing. Perseveration is the repetition of a particular behaviour or thought, rumination is the act of dwelling on negative thoughts or emotions. Ugh.

☺ There must surely be a happy medium between Mack's persevering and perseverating and my procrastinating and giving up.

Takeaways for Mack
- When he's 'stuck' on something, consider whether he's persevering or perseverating/ruminating.
- In either case, consider the downside of carrying on rather than taking a break or putting off finishing.

- Talk to Shonagh about any underlying anxiety that's causing negative perseverating.
- Use the chuck-it bucket.

Takeaways for me
- Look out for perseverating thoughts or behaviours and check with Mack what's going on in his head.

Uncertainty

19 February

To Auties, there's nothing worse than uncertainty, and this leads them to ask question after question and to research things to death. It drives their 'need to know'. Much as it drives the rest of us mad.

Uncertainty and the need to know become a big issue where health is involved, exacerbating Mack's medical anxiety. This means we need to do lots of homework before a medical appointment. Let's take, for example, the MRI. I mentioned before that Mack had done all his research so that he knew what to expect – what the machine looked like, how it worked, what it sounded like, how long it would take, etc. But that was only part of the picture. The first worry was whether we'd even get there in time. So we booked a room in the hotel beside the hospital for the night before and did a recce of the hospital grounds to find the right building/entrance and decide which car park to use. Even then, we had to get there half an hour early next morning.

I hadn't appreciated how important it is for an Autie to know exactly what to expect and when. Preparing for an appointment – of any kind – is like preparing for an exam.

The National Autistic Society stresses the importance of reducing anxiety around uncertainty, and suggests doing this, firstly, by ensuring the autistic person knows what to expect and, secondly, by gradually rather than suddenly exposing them to uncertain situations[20]. So I'm glad to hear we've been getting this right.

😳 Sometimes things change unexpectedly and, when this happens, it's important to have a back-up plan.

Fortunately, Mack excels at back-up plans! This could be something simple like checking out an alternative route in case of a problem with the preferred one. Or it could be something like having music or some other distraction to help cope with any delay. There was no back-up plan for suddenly finding you needed to be strapped into an MRI machine though, hence the "dignified meltdown" when that happened!

Now that I understand this aspect of autism, I'm astounded by how well Mack hid some of the anxieties I've unwittingly inflicted on him myself over the years. Simple things, like holidays even. Everyone, surely, looks forward to a sunny summer holiday – a well-deserved reward for a year's hard slog? You spend ages choosing a lovely place to go, then planning how to get there and what you'll see and do – I used to love it.

Mack seemed quite happy to play along for a good few years, but I do remember him voicing some hesitation. For example, as a business owner rather than an employee, he was anxious about being away from the office for any more than a week at a time. So holidays had to be short. Looking back, this was a bit of a hollow excuse given he was glued to his Blackberry (yes, we're going back a bit) day and night wherever he was. But he did *appear* to enjoy our holidays

---

[20] National Autistic Society (2018), Anxiety in autistic people. Accessed February 2023 at:
https://www.autism.org.uk/advice-and-guidance/professional-practice/anxiety-autism

in Lake Garda, Fuerteventura, Mijas, Madeira, Barcelona, Tenerife…

<<Yes, I did enjoy most of those holidays once we got there and I started to relax a bit. That generally took two or three days – I was so exhausted from having been working so hard that I didn't have energy to do much in the way of activities or exploring.

In retrospect though, I wonder if the exhaustion was as much to do with the holiday itself as overworking.

The worst thing was not knowing whether we'd get to the airport in time and then whether the flight would be on time – I find delays of any kind hard to handle – and airports and planes are such unpleasant places to have to hang around.

And there's the destination too. Going somewhere completely unfamiliar and facing the associated onslaught of sensory processing is pretty taxing to say the least – although I didn't understand that then.>>

Mack

20 February

Flying was also a bit of an issue. This puzzled me because Mack used to fly all over the world in his previous life – Singapore one week, Chicago or Boston the next, the odd hop to Bermuda and shuttling back and forth to London all the time. But he was definitely a nervous flyer and seemed to get a little worse with each successive holiday. His explanation was one too many scares – he was sure he'd used up his nine flying lives already.

> <<I don't think there was one specific incident I could put it down to – it was more of a cumulative thing.
>
> There was one flight that hit severe turbulence, and a guy who was sitting nearby and hadn't strapped himself in just about knocked himself out on the overhead bins. That was a horrible flight. I remember being on a plane that took off so sharply it almost scraped its tail on the ground. Another bumped the terminal building. And once, when we were coming in to land during bad weather, the winds were so bad the plane was *flapping*. I was *so* glad to get down!
>
> I think I already mentioned the plane with the explosive device that had to be detonated by the bomb squad. Yep, that was scary. It makes you think about the PanAm flight that came down in Lockerbie in 1988 – the horror is unimaginable.
>
> When you add scary and unpleasant flights to the sensory challenges and stresses involved in travelling by air, I can quite honestly say I'd rather face a dental extraction with no anaesthetic than have to do it again.>>
>
> Mack

Mack would be on tenterhooks for a good few days before setting off and then started dreading the return trip only halfway through the holiday. Eventually, I got to the point of thinking it just wasn't worth it.

We reached a compromise though – we could go on holiday if only he didn't have to fly. Game on. I'd miss basking in the sunshine, but so long as the temperature was reasonable and there was plenty of interest to see and do, I'd be happy enough. So our next holiday was to Bruges, because we could just nip over the channel from Rosyth to Zeebrugge. Nothing could be simpler. He definitely seemed a lot more relaxed on the ferry than on a flight, but strangely – well, not so strangely now that we know what we know now! – he didn't seem very chilled out during our time there which was disappointing.

My niece, Juliana, was getting married in Catalonia in 2013 and so that was to be our next holiday. For Mack, this was probably the greatest holiday hurdle he's ever faced. Our plans to go by train fell through when they decided to cancel the sleeper service to Barcelona with little or no warning, leaving us high and dry. So the restful trip we'd anticipated became a tortuous bumper-to-bumper dodgem drive from Edinburgh to Portsmouth, followed by a 24-hour ferry trip to Santander and then a slightly more relaxing day's meander (once beyond Bilbao) across the top of Spain on lovely, virtually empty motorway.

The party lasted the full week with thirty-odd people sharing a villa – a joy for any Autie, as you can imagine – and then we faced the equally tortuous return trip. It was a lovely wedding, and everyone had a wonderful time, but the person I took home with me at the end of the week was an empty shell. A mere ghost of a man who could no longer string two words together!

We've only attempted two foreign holidays since, both much smaller undertakings, travelling by car and ferry to West Flanders in Belgium and Picardy in France. And although Mack didn't have to face flights or stay in a party villa, he still found it hard. At least we both understand why now.

So, if we ever decide to go on holiday again, here's what we'll do:

- Choose a quiet destination and go at a quiet time.
- Don't just look at a guidebook or the internet; explore the place thoroughly using Google street view – or go to a place we've been before.
- Travel by car and ferry and stay in secluded, self-catering accommodation.
- Build in sufficient psych-up and recuperation time for both the holiday and any planned excursions.
- Use the full kit'n caboodle of the sensory emergency kit as required.

Hopefully, if we can reduce the anxiety and sensory overload in this way, Mack can finally know what it's like to *enjoy* a holiday rather than endure it.

😕 **We need to apply all these lessons to daily life.**

Takeaways for Mack
- Keep planning and researching to control any anxiety and reduce uncertainty.
- Don't worry about what other people think – his own wellbeing is more important than other people's perceptions.

Takeaways for me
- To ease the load on Mack, start thinking the same way – planning, researching, preparing, spacing things out and having back-up plans. Ugh.

21 February

Having to think ventures through carefully and considerately sounds a little onerous, but there *is* a silver lining to Mack's need to understand anything and everything.

If I want to know something but can't be bothered finding out about it for myself, the chances are high that he'll already know the answer. It's certainly worth checking. While he may not remember what we agreed to have for dinner, or the plot of a film we've seen several times, he can retain huge amounts of useless and sometimes use*ful* facts.

And if there's something he doesn't already know, he's not long finding out. For example, during a conversation recently, my mother mentioned a great uncle who bred dogs in America and brought them over here to sell in the 1960s and 70s. Mack asked a few questions – "What was his name?", "What kind of dogs?", "Where in America?" The uncle's first name we couldn't remember, and we even argued over the spelling of his surname. The dogs apparently were sheepdogs, and I remembered he lived in Pottersville from having done a little dead rellie research a few years ago. "Found him!" Mack said a minute or two later, as he showed us photos on his phone of Great Uncle Lawrie and his border collies in a local paper from the 1970s.

He's not so good at wait and see though. Mack: "Annuity rates up? Buy now!" Me: "But I think they might go higher yet…" But *might* means uncertainty, and that's excruciating.

Mack: "I think we should buy that last house we saw." Me: "But you hated it!" Mack: "Well, yeah, but I've thought about it more and I'm sure it'll be fine…" Yes, he'd rather buy a house he didn't like than face weeks and months of unsettling house-hunting.

Me: "I should probably change my car next year." Mack, half an hour later: "I've found you the perfect car, and we can be there in 40 minutes." Actually, there could be a few explanations for that one. Uncertainty – he can't stand not knowing if and when I'll change my car or what I might replace it with. Listening – he only heard 'change my car'. Or it could just be his desperate need to both start and finish!

Suddenly changing plans on him or subverting his expectations can definitely cause a wobbly, if not an out-and-out meltdown. Examples I've brushed on already include that first abortive MRI appointment and when our travel plans for the Catalonia trip went belly up.

More recently, the cancer coordinator called to give Mack a date for his operation. We'd been led to expect this would happen in April (as the waiting list was four months at the time of agreeing to this treatment), but the date proposed was 21 March. Way too soon for his Autie mind to be prepared for. And only one week after the scheduled appointment to discuss the procedure and coping mechanisms to (a) get him there in the first place and (b) get him through it. Yep, there was no way that was happening. Sadly, the poor coordinator hadn't 'got the memo' about his autism.

Empathy

23 February

We're watching TV, most likely the news, and there's a story about someone who has said or done something foolish or reckless or greedy maybe. If you're a kind person, you might feel a bit sorry for them – that's if you have any feelings about it one way or the other. Mack's more likely to go off on one and start ranting at the TV. He does that a lot.

Is he showing a lack of empathy? I don't think that's it. In any case, it's a myth that Auties don't feel empathy, it's just that they vary in the way they experience and express it.

With Mack, I sometimes wonder if the empathy he shows depends on how well he knows and cares about the person – or respects or relates to them. As I mentioned before, he would do anything for his family and friends and would defend them to the ends of the earth. Albeit that would be a bit stressy!

> <<Although Dad was a distant figure in my early life as he was always working, he was my 'place of safety' during a tortuous childhood, and he became a very good friend in later life. He hid and managed my poor mother's Alzheimer's successfully for some considerable time before we realised what was going on and that he really needed help. I couldn't bear to think how hard it was for him both physically and emotionally.
>
> After a while, he wasn't able to leave my mother alone even for the time it took to cook something simple, so as a family we put in

place as much support as we could get and spent our weekends batch-cooking all their meals so the carers could simply nuke them.

Over the next year or two, my sister Eilidh and I hared back and forth along the motorway between Edinburgh and Glasgow, responding to SOSs at all times of the day or night. We'd often be halfway there only to receive a call standing us down again. It was hard-going, but I'd never not have been there for him.>>

Mack

Mack often stops and speaks to people begging on the street. They're usually strangers but, as it turns out, not always.

He was walking along George Street in Edinburgh one day, past a chap who was sitting on a slightly grubby sleeping bag with the obligatory little sign and cap. The face rang a bell, and then a little wave of horror and a cold sweat swept over Mack as he placed the man: a former banking colleague, Geoff.

Turns out his life had simply gone sideways – whether resulting in depression or as a result of depression I can no longer recall – it's a vicious circle after all. But he'd lost everything along the way – wife, family, friends, job, home… And with no one left to spot the signs of his mental illness or care enough to get him any help, he found himself living on the streets.

That said, he'd become accustomed to his new life and seemed quite content. His slightly grubby sleeping bag was his most prized possession – not some cheap bit of tat, but the best the local mountaineering shop had to offer.

<<There but for the grace of God…

I was *so* lucky not to reach that point. But I did sleep in my car for a while after giving up on my first marriage. And I did live on baked beans and cheap wine for some time after that. I know what it's like to suddenly find yourself not only penniless but laden with mounting debt and so depressed you've lost the will to face the light of day.

So I don't judge others who, like Geoff, find themselves reduced to sitting on the streets. Behind every single beggar there's a story, and a little compassion goes a long way – after all, you're only one piece of bad luck away from being there yourself.>>

Mack

☉ **An autistic person's empathy, based on instincts and involuntary responses to other people's emotions, can be strong and even overwhelming.**

A while back, my sister Marnie and her partner Grady had some problems with the drainage on their property – now all sorted, thankfully. Marnie is generally a very chilled-out person, but the worry had her on the ceiling, and if she could have put the house on the market the very next day, she probably would have.

Mack's reaction was to research the problem for hours and suggest all sorts of solutions. From ordering new fuses for their septic tank, to digging out an old hose of his own to help pump the water away, to giving Marnie a selection of calm-me-down remedies, he couldn't do enough to help. When, to top it all, he gave her a sandless sandbag, Marnie was moved to tears which instantly resulted in his own eyes welling up!

So his empathy for those he cares about is clear. But I still struggled to understand his lack of empathy for those he rants at on TV, until I stumbled on an old article that was talking about autism and judgement, recounting research conducted by MIT[21].

In this study, people were asked to rate the morality of a woman who'd made coffee for a visitor using white powder from a bowl labelled 'sugar', but which turned out to be poison. The visitor died. While neurotypical people don't usually judge someone's behaviour immoral if they acted with good intentions but on bad information, the research found that people with what used to be called 'high-functioning autism' were more likely to judge the poisoner harshly.

Could it simply be that the news stories about the people who have said or done the foolish or reckless or greedy things are offending Mack's sense of morality? Note to self: next time, pay more attention to what the person has done to trigger the rant.

<<Ranting?! I'm merely expressing an opinion…!>>

Mack

---

[21] Los Angeles Times (2011), Autism's moral judgment gap explored. Accessed February 2023 at:
https://www.latimes.com/health/la-xpm-2011-jan-31-la-heb-autism-judgment-20110131-story.html

24 February

OK, here's another thing. Two people are squabbling over the TV remote, unable to agree on what to watch. One of them is an Autie, the other's not.

Viewer one enjoys *Dragon's Den*, a show where entrepreneurs give a short pitch to win investment monies from the dragons, and the dragons interrogate them brutally on their business plan. Viewer two hates the show – they feel every agony the entrepreneurs are going through. It's very stressful, which makes it seriously unpleasant to watch.

Next up, they're choosing between two films, one of which they've both seen and enjoyed many times. The other doesn't sound familiar – could be good, could be awful. Viewer one is happy to watch either, but viewer two would rather see the first film for the umpteenth time than risk enduring another ghastly viewing experience.

Given what we now understand about how Auties experience stress and anxiety – and about repetitive behaviours and the importance of familiarity as opposed to the unexpected – the smart money's on viewer two being the Autie, right?

Nope. *Mack* is viewer one; *I'm* the one who can't bear to watch the stress these dragons put the entrepreneurs through. *I'm* the one who would prefer to see the same film again and again and again rather than endure a couple of hours of monotony or worse. (Yes, I know, I should revisit that AQ test again!)

I've challenged Mack about this – well, about *Dragon's Den* specifically, wanting to understand why he doesn't feel the entrepreneurs' stress. Having been in a similar situation himself when seeking venture capital for starting up his own business, I'd have thought he'd really feel for them.

> <<I'm just interested in the investment side of things – the business, how it operates, the ideas, the opportunities, the gaps. I don't feel empathy for them at all because they should know what to expect and be prepared. If they're not, it's their own fault.>>
>
> Mack

Oh. Harsh. But it sheds some light on this anomaly – he's not relating to the people at all, he's dispassionately assessing the business opportunities and remaining objective. For Mack, it's simply all about black and white facts and figures. I wish I could dissociate like that!

But this would seem to support the theory that Mack keeps his empathy for people he knows, cares about and/or respects or relates to.

According to my investigations, true empathy happens on three levels – thoughts, feelings and actions. Your thoughts reflect your ability to put yourself in another person's shoes. Your feelings reflect your ability to experience, at least to an extent, the other person's emotions – so when they cry you find yourself crying too. Your actions reflect what you do to help, given your understanding of the person's needs in the circumstances – from giving them a simple hug or listening ear to making suggestions or lending practical support of some kind.

😕 **Empathy is a conscious choice. For people you care about it makes sense that you'd go all the way, but it would be too overwhelming to take on the cares of the**

world so, for your own mental wellbeing, you need to strike a balance.

Takeaways for Mack
- Try to care for himself at least half as much as he does for others who matter to him.

Takeaways for me
- As Mack has the ability to care too much, his lack of empathy towards people he doesn't know and has never met is healthy – and in fact very important for his wellbeing.

Integrity

27 February

You're out for a walk in the country and a £10 note flutters across your path. There's not a soul in sight. What do you do? The way I see it, there's no way of knowing who might have lost it and nowhere to hand it in, so I'll give it a good home without a second thought. Not Mack. It would burn a hole in his conscience because he knows it's not his, and he'd donate it to the nearest charity as fast as he possibly could.

If someone gives him change of £10 instead of £5, he'll immediately hand back the extra fiver. If he receives a delivery of something better and more expensive than the item he actually ordered, he'll call to return it right away. And if he's promised to do something, he'll move heaven and earth to make sure he can do it.

Autism? Upbringing? A bit of both?

Further research shows that Auties often have a strong moral code – a deep sense of moral justice and fairness. They're more likely to be selfless and to show integrity in their moral values than neurotypical people. Sadly, this can often make their lives harder.

Early in his career, Mack was distressed to discover unethical behaviour at a senior level in the department he was working in. His attempts to call it out resulted in him being sent to the banking equivalent of Siberia. He moved on.

A decade later, something similar happened and, unable to do anything from within the organisation, he felt he had no option but to blow the whistle to the regulator. This set his career back for a second time.

In yet another company several years after that, he began to suspect serious wrongdoing and started asking questions. Too many questions. And he hadn't uncovered sufficient evidence to do anything about it before he was effectively shown the door. Yep, this is beginning to sound very much like 'repetitive behaviour'!

> <<I know it's not career enhancing. Nor it is understood by those on the receiving end, but it's important. I can't stand people taking advantage or ripping others off – it's just not right.
>
> On the upside, I've worked with many firms who have shown the highest levels of integrity and that's been rewarding. And much less stressful!>>
>
> Mack

😯 Autistic people have a desire and tendency to follow rules and to tell the truth – even if it's not tactful or in their own interests.

This tendency to follow rules played a good part in Mack's ultimate choice of career – as I'd concluded earlier. While he started in banking and spent a while as a systems analyst, he then gravitated towards financial services compliance. End-to-end rules and regulations designed to fry the average brain – who wouldn't want to do that?

Mack had an employee who after some personal struggles turned quietly to drink to try and cope. On discovering this, Mack supported them in every way he could, including giving them time off and paying out of his own pocket for counselling – at a time when he was struggling to make ends meet himself. This seemed to help. But a year or two later things got worse again and came to a head following a drunken incident at the office after hours.

Mack found himself in a terrible position – torn between compassion for his employee and loyalty to his business and clients, whose confidentiality or data protection were likely to be put at risk unless he took action.

Anyone else would have fired the employee for gross misconduct. Instead, Mack offered redundancy, putting the interests of both the employee and his clients well above his own.

This is in stark contrast to a previous occasion when he had to fire someone. Under compliance rules, you have to declare gifts you're given over a certain value to be sure your integrity isn't compromised and that you're not influenced by them in any way. Essentially, you're not supposed to accept bribes. Anyway, this employee declared a Christmas hamper he was given, but didn't declare the car it was in the boot of. Obviously, Mack had absolutely no qualms about that one.

>><<Dad couldn't stand people stealing or manipulating either. The organisation he worked for had a listed building of historical significance to Glasgow. It was furnished with handcrafted period pieces which were relevant to the building, its history and the city. During renovations, the board room table and all the chairs, each of which represented a trade or craft in the Glasgow area, were placed into storage.

By sheer chance, Dad had to attend a senior board director's house to pick him up for an inspection of some outlying properties and noticed that 10 of the chairs were now sitting around the dining room table. He was incandescent. The director was given an ultimatum – to return the chairs immediately or a call would be made to the police. The chairs were eventually returned, but Dad was made redundant within three months.>>

Mack

Like son like father it would seem. So, is Mack's sense of integrity as much to do with upbringing as his autism, or do we think maybe father Tam was an Autie too? Answers on a postcard.

☺ **You can learn integrity, but if it's part of who you are, you can't switch it off.**

Takeaways for Mack
- Remember not everyone has a moral compass as powerful as his.
- Remember too that people make genuine mistakes and often feel the need to cover them up – it's worth more research before reaching a damning conclusion.

Takeaways for me
- Let him do the research.

Enthusiasms and special interests

28 February

Kind people call Auties' particular interests passions; the more exasperated call them obsessions. Enthusiasms seems more appropriate for Mack, although I blush to say it because I'm just as bad myself! As I said, I very much fear I'm on the cusp.

If I find a *really* good book for example, it would take something like a fire to stop me reading before I get to the end – even if it takes till 5am! And then there's dead rellie hunting (aka genealogy), drawing, writing this. Fully absorbing for a while, but eventually I reach a point of losing interest – usually once something or someone distracts me. (But let's hope I *do* manage to finish this.)

Mack seems to have always been driven by a desire to prove himself – to be the very best he can be at whatever he chooses to do. I don't mean DIY – he's great at getting things done but finesse isn't really his thing! At work though, he had to do the best job possible and his reputation was hugely important to him. That meant he was never off duty – taking calls and sending emails at all times of the day or night. He didn't understand the concept of a holiday.

His 'thing' for cars might be considered an enthusiasm – 29 cars in 22 years surely *must* come under at least one autism heading. And he can identify the issue behind every clunk, ping, squeak, squeal and groan a car can make.

> <<Until work became all-consuming, I used to have a lot of interests.
>
> Outside of school or work and evening classes, I taught violin and, after qualifying at

16, I taught speech and drama for a while too. I played badminton once a week, did a lot of road cycling and played golf every chance I could get. I was always an avid reader and piano player. I also played the viola in school and theatre orchestras and was an active member of the Rotaract which I joined at 18.

From my mid-twenties, family commitments took up more of my time so my main focus – or interest – became my work. Although I was always motivated to be the best I could be, whatever the context, it was more rewarding when I found a niche that satisfied my desire to research and problem-solve within a well-regulated environment.>>

Mack

Apart from work, cars and music, Mack's enthusiasms seem to be short term. At first glance, this doesn't sound as though it fits the stereotypical autistic profile, which includes a 'special interest' of narrow and intense focus. That said, it's clear that every Autie is different – each ticking different boxes to different degrees. For Mack, I'd say it's more about 'special projects' than special interests. He always has to have a project on the go, and during that project he's almost obsessed by it. (Yes, I know, pot kettle black.)

For example, and off the top of my head, here are just some of his pet projects over the last three years – most of which were bolthole undertakings. Let me see…

- Upgrading the electrics in the entire place having uncovered some hidden horrors.
- Upgrading the garage to turn it into his ideal man cave.

- Creating a downstairs shower room for the convenience of guests.
- Creating a pathway of sleepers through a steep banking to make gardening easier.
- Rebuilding his classic car.
- Building the 'car stopper' – a solid stone boundary wall to stop speeding cars from careering off the road and into the fishpond (which *has* happened).
- Building and fitting out his 'summer house'.
- Making a violin from scratch for son Stuart's 30th birthday.
- Extending the patio and building the potting shed.
- Dividing the living room into two to create a small bedroom and add value to the property.
- Researching prostate cancer and its treatments.
- Creating a workshop in the derelict outhouse…

Some of these schemes he undertook because, whether he enjoyed the work or not, he enjoyed the outcome – the garage, the car, the summer house. But others he undertook because of an underlying concern. For example, if we didn't address the electrics, the building would burn down and "we'd be crispy duck".

Each of the projects was all-consuming at the time and entailed quite a bit of perseverance.

😮 **Some special interests are transient rather than lifelong, and there are clear benefits in having special interests.**

Many of the older articles I found while researching special interests talked about them in negative language. For example, 'obsessions', 'restricted interests', 'avoidance activities'. But more recently, the focus has moved to the rewards and benefits.

Such interests can build self-confidence and be a springboard for learning. You can become an expert in your field of interest, which could make you a go-to person on the subject, and it can also give you a platform for social interaction. Many Auties make a career out of their area of expertise – Albert Einstein, Chris Packham, Elon Musk.

In Mack's case, the combination of research and perseverance involved in a project or enthusiasm also means getting things done and getting them done right. So even when he's not doing a job himself – for example, where he needs the skill and experience of a specialist tradesman – he'll know what needs to be done, understand how best to do it and be able to supervise the work to ensure it's completed to his satisfaction.

Turns out Mack's not the only one whose enthusiasms are transient, and a study of nearly 2,000 autistic kids in 2020 showed they had an average of nine special interests at a time[22].

>   <<I built a violin because I wanted to give Stuart something personal, meaningful. Something he could look back on and think 'Dad made that for me.' I also hoped he might play it from time to time as he used to be a good violinist himself, but life tends to get in the way of small pleasures like that.
>
>   I'd repaired violins before but never attempted to build one from a blank piece of wood. It was a challenge, and I like a

---

[22] Spectrum (2021), The benefits of special interests in autism. Accessed February 2023 at:
https://www.spectrumnews.org/features/deep-dive/the-benefits-of-special-interests-in-autism

challenge. I discovered new skills and relearned old ones Dad had taught me many years ago. Beyond a small investment in wood and strings, the rest was just time and effort. There was an element of frustration of course, such as in trying to learn tricky new techniques, but that's the virtue of YouTube – you can watch other people doing the same or a similar task which is a great way to learn. That was particularly helpful for carving and fixing the neck.

However, I was having a problem getting the sound posts and blocks for these in the right position and couldn't find anything showing that. Happily, it turned out that my pest controller pal Declan used to work in his grandad's violin workshop years ago, so he was able to give me a great steer. No, I wasn't boring him senseless about my 'special interest of the moment'! He'd just casually asked me what I was up to, and I was happy to tell him.

I actually felt a massive sense of joy when I'd finished it – with days to spare. It looked good, it worked, it sounded beautiful and will only get better with age.>>

Mack

Following a pointer from Number 6, a little further digging on the subject of interests led me to monotropism. If you're monotropic, you tend to focus more of your attention on fewer things at any one time. As a result, you might miss things that are happening outside of an "attention tunnel", and moving from one tunnel to another can be hard and take a lot of energy. Or, as better explained by monotropism.org, "Monotropic minds tend to have their attention pulled more strongly towards a smaller number of interests at any given time, leaving fewer resources for other processes."[23]

Ah, that seems to describe both of us pretty well!

1 March

Now that Mack's retiring, he'll have a lot more spare time on his hands which is a concern – the last thing we need is for him to be bored and simply find things to worry about. We need to make sure his extra time is spent enjoyably, and to do that, we need to identify a bunch of enjoyable – and given his current state of health, less strenuous – things for him to do!

Where to begin? Some of the ideas he's started kicking around already include: photography – which he's done as a money-making hobby before; cooking – he used to rustle up some tasty dishes before gastro limitations took the shine out of it; gardening – there's plenty of that needing done at the bolthole and it's something he certainly *used* to enjoy.

Is there still a demand for repairing violins? Tutoring? Mentoring?

Mack used to find charity work very rewarding, so it would be great to get back into that. Say, looking for volunteering opportunities without too much in the way of social contact and sensory challenges.

Or he could perhaps get involved in helping others to start up their own businesses – he's actually done a little of that

---

[23] Monotropism (2023), Welcome. Accessed February 2023 at: **https://monotropism.org**

incidentally over the past few years. Or even start up a small online, stress-free business of his own.

😜 **Mack definitely needs something to keep him entertained and out of trouble while I'm still working!**

Takeaways for Mack
- Do only projects that will be fun or satisfying – we can get help to do necessary and stressy ones, and any others he can consign to the chuck-it bucket.
- Try to slow down the pace out of respect for his ageing bones. A project really *doesn't* need to be done all at once or in a day.

Takeaways for me
- Keep steering him towards positive, rewarding and enjoyable activities and projects.

Gifts

2 March

It seems that many Auties are gifted in some way or another. But it's hard to know where the line is between having become very good at something through dedication or enthusiasm and having a gift – an exceptional natural ability or talent.

Mack's incredible visual (photographic) memory is an aspect of his autism, but it could also be considered a gift as it's an ability he's never had to work at and it's undoubtedly helped him in his career.

He's also pretty bright, having scored an IQ of 147 when tested as a child. Again, that's not something you have to work at, but is it a gift? According to my investigations, yes. If you have an IQ level of 130 or higher, which falls within the top 2% of the population, you're considered to be gifted. It can't harm your life chances to be smart, but I do wonder if what you gain on the swings of IQ, you lose on the roundabouts of common sense!

And then there's the music.

Mack first started playing piano at around five years old. However, he wasn't a big fan of his teacher who seemed to be into nothing but scales, and so he only stuck at it for about three years. The lessons, that is. He continued to play for his own enjoyment after that, albeit periodically.

Then, when he started at the high school aged nine, he was given his first violin. I'm not clear whether this was because he particularly wanted to take up a string instrument, or because it was a great way of getting out of games – as PE classes used to be called – but he certainly liked his violin teacher a lot better than he'd liked his piano teacher.

At age 11 the lessons stopped but, with a quick switch from violin to viola, the playing continued as he earned himself a spot in the school orchestra. A year later, he joined the Glasgow schools' orchestras as well, working his way up from the third orchestra to the first over the next three years.

Why the switch to viola? This was essentially because he inherited the most colossal pair of hands from his maternal grandfather. Playing the smaller instrument became trickier as they grew into full sized spades, so viola made sense. Fortunately, they didn't *keep* growing or he would have had to try the double bass next.

At 15, Mack started to play for theatre orchestras from time to time, firstly just standing in for his tutor on occasions when *he* wasn't free to play, but soon earning spots in his own right. He also took up the saxophone for a couple of years.

Sadly, Mack followed advice to get a 'proper job' on leaving school rather than becoming a musician, but I know he's always regretted it and wondered where that other path may have taken him. Given how good music is for the soul, I suspect he may have led a happier life.

>><<Yehudi Menuhin was my childhood hero. He's widely considered one of the greatest violinists of the 20th century, and I was lucky enough not only to have met him once but to have actually played with him for a little while as a 14-year-old!

I had gone to listen to a regional heat of Young Musician of the Year, straight after I'd been at an orchestra rehearsal. I didn't realise it was Yehudi Menuhin I was sitting next to until he touched my arm and asked if I could play a specific two-part piece – he'd noticed I had my viola with me. He said he was looking for someone to warm up with before he was due to play it on stage; and if I could spare half an hour, did I want to play the other part for him. It was amazing, and I came away with so many tips!

What's more, he also asked me to turn the pages for him on stage during the performance. Sadly, I was so starstruck that I fluffed a turn when I was up there, only to receive a crack of the bow across the paper! But meeting and playing with him is an experience I've always prized and will never forget – he truly was an inspiration.>>

Mack

After leaving school, Mack continued to play the viola for several years in theatre orchestras, the earnings from which made his bank salary look very miserly. But the demands of his day job, life, and studying for professional qualifications gradually squeezed out the time he had for pleasures like this.

Although he never played music professionally again, Mack does still play the piano at home. He doesn't use sheet music – he seems to just pick up and play everything by ear – and he won't play in front of people. But it's something that relaxes him and it definitely lifts his mood.

3 March

😮 **Autism is often associated with significant musical abilities, and it's been shown that music can reduce stress and anxiety levels.**

Mack has in fact used music to help him through stressful events before. Before being diagnosed, I mean. It's one of the things that's helped him during dental appointments – a good piece of music at high volume through the AirPods is a great way to drown out the sound of the drill. Sorry, Mr Whizzy.

My investigations tell me that autism and giftedness can go hand in hand, although one doesn't necessarily imply the other. Gifted kids and Auties with high IQs do seem to have a lot in common though. For example:

- They're quick to learn but get bored easily so need stimulation and challenge.
- They have good memories and creative approaches to solving complex problems.
- They can feel things more intensely, be a little different or difficult and find themselves socially excluded.
- They often underachieve in formal education through anxiety, lack of interest in the subjects or because they're continually distracted by things that are more important to them.

Yep, that sounds like Mack.

> <<I do remember being a bit bored at primary school – although surely everyone must have felt that occasionally, especially when the teacher was covering a subject that didn't interest you or that you already knew about. But I believe I was considered 'disruptive'

and I know the teachers didn't like me very much because of that.

Only the headmistress thought to do anything about it though. She suggested to my parents while I was in primary four that they try to get me into a selective grammar school, which I would find more challenging. And, I suspect, because it would get me out of their hair! I duly sat the entrance test to gain admission, and joined at the beginning of the next academic year when I was nine.

Although I was pleased to get in, it was a bit of a culture shock. Suddenly, I wasn't the brightest pupil anymore – they were all smart kids there. And there was nothing in the way of 'pastoral care' – quite the opposite in fact. The school believed in survival of the fittest and bullying was not only rife but blatantly ignored by the staff who thought that was the kind of thing that 'made you a man'.

For a variety of reasons, it's fair to say I underachieved academically, but it wasn't all bad. I'd never have had the same opportunities in music or to join the cadets had I gone anywhere else, and those are precious memories.>>

Mack

I began this journey wondering how Mack could have hidden his autism for 63 years, but some of the articles I've read suggest that a gifted autistic person is very likely to be able to hide his or her difficulties and indeed differences quite successfully and for a long time. A combination of a high IQ and an aptitude for masking will certainly have helped him do that.

😐 **It's never too late to enjoy a gift.**

Takeaways for Mack
- Keep playing the piano, and why not dig out the viola too?
- Add listening to music to the toolbox, alongside counting, breathing, time-outs, etc.

Takeaways for me
- Keep encouraging him to play, and also to listen to music at home or in the car more often.

Clumsiness

4 March

We christened them the suicide steps because they were dangerously steep and uneven, but he fell down them anyway, tearing his Achilles. I warned him not to use those ladders – they looked well iffy. But I foolishly let him out of my sight and half an hour later we were in A&E with three broken ribs. And just the other week he managed to knock over and smash a crystal vase, a breakfast bowl and an electric hotplate in three separate incidents.

Yep, clumsiness is a 'thing' too. Mack is very good at health and safety for others – I'm endlessly being lectured on doing things carefully, but it's very much a case 'don't do as I do, do as I tell you'. We have a shed full of safety gear and a cabinet full of first aid stuff – guess which is used the most? Yes, that's a rhetorical question.

The absolute worst example of Mack's clumsiness, or lack of coordination, would be an episode during his childhood when he and his father were fishing. The story is too gory to tell. Let's just say – turn away if you're squeamish – that it wasn't a fish he caught that day and that his father Tam lost the sight in his right eye.

> <<It was beyond horrific, seeing Dad with a hook (a three-pronged mackerel lure) in his eye. But he was amazing.
>
> You might expect someone to scream or at least to panic and shout or swear in that situation, but he was so incredibly calm. He didn't say a word the whole time, while we ran about like headless chickens, bundling him into the car and racing to the hospital.

> Even afterwards, when it was clear he'd never get his sight back, he didn't breathe a single word of censure or reproach. Ever.
>
> I don't have the words to describe how I feel about the way he coped with that incident and its repercussions – 'respect' just doesn't cut it. I couldn't be prouder to have had him as a father – and to have had such a wonderful example of how to be a father myself one day. This horrific episode brought us closer and made for a lifelong friendship.>>
>
> Mack

The bit about this story that gives me pause for thought now is how calmly Tam took it. Autism is genetic, isn't it? Is it possible that Tam could have gone undiagnosed for 91 years and that what Mack's describing is actually a meltdown of the 'becoming totally passive and playing dead' variety? I guess we'll never know.

Mack used to play badminton pretty well, long before I knew him, so he must have *some* coordination. But you wouldn't know it to see him with a golf club. The odds would be fairly even between landing a hole in one or a hole in the clubhouse window. Yes, *duck!* if you see him with any kind of an implement.

Oh yes – he's got quite a history of window-breaking. As a 10-year-old, he had a particularly notable spate of it. First, he was playing golf in his garden – using real golf balls against explicit instructions – and pitched a ball straight through the dining room window which ricocheted off the rear wall and back out through a different pane. A couple of days later, in a strop with his very little sister, he hurled a toy gun across the room which somehow catapulted through the living room window. And a week or so after that, when he found himself locked out of the house, he tried to get in via the bathroom window, but fell through, breaking the glass and knackering the toilet seat in the process. The glazier is reputed to have made some crack about Beirut by the time he'd made this third visit!

I asked Mack if he'd ever done himself any serious harm (that I didn't already know about) through his clumsiness, and he admitted to having broken his arm tripping through a school doorway as a kid. He chipped his ulna and broke the radius. The radius was sticking through the skin and compromising his circulation, so the rugby coach popped it back into place, bound his arm and put it in a sling. Then they simply sent him home. That was a trip that took an hour and a half by foot and train, and only then was he taken to hospital to get his arm reset. Glad I didn't go to *that* school, but they're made of hard stuff, Weegies!

☺ **Many autistic people are accident prone – something to do with the wiring responsible for motor function.**

<<As a kid, I'd put my hand on the centre pillar of the car, close the door, and wonder why it hurt! Often you get so absorbed in something that you lose sight of peripheral risks...>>

Mack

He made that sound like past history, didn't he? But he did exactly the same thing only a few days ago, dislocating a little finger. Although it clicked back into place, that blackened nail is definitely not going to survive much longer. And only last night he almost glassed himself when he tripped up the stairs carrying a drink of water.

5 March

I wonder if there's anything in his comment about getting so absorbed in something that you don't notice risks. Back to Google…

OK, it looks like the answer is proprioception – one of those extra three sensory systems that I knew nothing about before researching autism. This is the one that's to do with movement. Or more specifically, your perception of your own movement and where bits of you are in relation to everything else. This is something that's controlled by the nerves in your body and the way they send messages.

So this is what they meant about the wiring responsible for motor function!

I keep coming across references to 'locating your body in space', which conjures up images of the starship Enterprise again. Well, these are certainly new frontiers for me. But what they mean is that proprioception is what tells us where our head and limbs are in relation to one another as well as where they begin and end. So I guess this is how I know that both my hands are on the keyboard and my feet are on the floor.

It's what allows us to perceive the world outside of our minds and how we're interacting with it. Without it, we may not know whether we're sitting, standing or moving. And it's not just about knowing *where* our body bits are, proprioception also tells us the extent to which our body bits need to interact with other things. For example, how hard to press the buttons on the keyboard. And it then controls or at least oversees those movements – I'm a bit woolly on the science around that bit, but I believe that's the gist of it. Oh, and it also measures and perceives distance, so that's how I know how far to reach when I want to click the mouse.

Ta-da! We've found the explanation for clumsiness. If your proprioception isn't up to scratch, you're going to be a bit of a hazard, to yourself and very probably others too!

What's particularly interesting – especially in light of Mack's comment earlier – is that Auties can show incredible dexterity when concentrating. Which they must have to do to play a musical instrument well. And they can also perform delicate operations or circus tricks but still trip over their own feet afterwards.

While it's perfectly possible to undertake a dextrous activity by focusing intently on it, someone with poor proprioception can't sustain this level of concentration indefinitely. Seems a bit unfair that Auties have to work so hard on this when the rest of us can do dexterity without even thinking about it.

So can anything be done to reduce clumsiness? For a vintage Autie, it seems unlikely, although there are suggestions that you can improve your sensory integration by doing balance and motion activities. Cycling, dancing, a bit of tai-chi maybe. Varifocal glasses certainly don't help.

We touched on balance under sensory sensitivity when I mentioned that walking on fractionally sloping floors made Mack feel woozy. And we noted when we first came across the three extra sensory systems that the vestibular one was responsible for balance. It looks as though, if your vestibular system doesn't work well, it affects your sense of balance and body control – which suggests this might play a little part in clumsiness too. It could explain Mack's penchant for falling off ladders, for example. But if your balance is affected, you're likely to get travel or motion sickness too.

Hmm, I'm not very sure what to make of this, because Mack doesn't seem to get sea sick even on pretty rough ferry crossings. He won't go on fairground rides such as the waltzers, but there could be many explanations for that...

OK, on balance (sorry!), and despite his ladder issue, I think Mack's clumsiness is due to proprioception rather than a dodgy sense of balance. Wouldn't being able to tell when a floor's off-level support that conclusion?

Having found the explanation for clumsiness, I realise we should have covered this under sensory sensitivity. Sorry about that – didn't see this one coming, such is the nature of taking a journaling approach to our investigations!

☹ **Mack's clumsiness could be hard to do anything about unless I put him in a playpen!**

Takeaways for Mack
- Be more careful. Yeah, right.
- Try some balance and motion exercises, at least until he's well enough to take up cycling again.
- Put the lights on, i.e. stop blundering about in the dark.

Takeaways for me
- Never leave him alone with a chainsaw, mandoline slicer or sharp knives! Although I'd sussed that one out long ago.

> <<The upside of my being safety conscious is that a first aid kit is never far away. This, together with a bit of first aid training – albeit from thirty-odd years back – has come in exceptionally handy over the years. And not just when I've injured myself, but when others have hit the buffers too.

When Stuart was a kid, he fell into a dead faint. He seemed to have stopped breathing completely. Thankfully, I knew just what to do to bring him back round.

I've had to deal with many injuries I've inflicted on myself over the years through misjudgement or clumsiness. The bloodiest incident happened when I was trying to repair a shed window – a sheet of glass slipped like a guillotine and went through my wrist. I had to extract it and sort myself out single-handed.

Way back in my banking days, a lady colleague had a heart attack. The ambulance didn't turn up – I can't remember what happened there – but we bundled her into a borrowed car and I got her to hospital fast with the help of a police escort!

I've also been able to help out at a couple of car crashes because I've always carried a first aid kit in the car.

More recently, Halle had a bad asthma attack while visiting and her inhaler was having no effect. I was able to give her a slug of oxygen which did the trick.>>

Mack

Punctuality

6 March

I get a little stressed if I think I'm going to be late, but I prefer to be just in time rather than too early. Not Mack.

This morning, a glazier was coming at 8am to fix a window problem; Mack set his alarm for 6.30am. Ugh. For his face-to-face appointments with Number 6, we had to be outside 40 minutes early – despite the astronomical cost of parking in the centre of Edinburgh. To be fair, if he has an appointment in a more familiar place he goes to more often, 20 minutes is fine. In the days when he used to fly, if we were supposed to check in for a noon flight at 10am, we'd need to be there by 8am if not sooner. I quickly learned never to book a morning flight!

After 20-odd years of this, I'm used to it. What caught me off guard more recently was discovering that being unexpectedly called *early* to start an appointment could induce a panic attack. That was for a meeting with Number 6 so, on the bright side, they're probably used to it.

However, I can recall at least one occasion where a slight blunder with timing caused a bit of a flip-out...

>><<It was 2014, one hundred years on from the beginning of the first world war, and Shonagh suggested we take a trip to visit Ypres and the battlefields of West Flanders. A short hop over the channel, no flying involved. I thought: OK, why not?

>>Sadly, the Rosyth ferry wasn't running anymore so we had to go all the way to Hull in England, but I'd done my research so knew

how long it would take to get there and had planned the route. But Shonagh had made the bookings and I took her word for it that the ferry departed at 5pm on the Sunday. That would have been 20 July. I figured that if we left home at 9am, we'd make it in plenty time, even allowing for a couple of breaks.

So Saturday was to be spent packing. It must have been early afternoon before I asked where the tickets were so that I could put all the documents together with the passports for the trip. A quick glance at them confirmed, yep, 5pm… On *Saturday 19* July! I can't even begin to describe how stressful that was – I'm going hot and cold at the memory!>>

Mack

Oops, mea culpa. Hope that didn't exacerbate his Autie issues. Thankfully, we were able to rebook the outward trip for the following day, albeit at a whopping extra cost.

I asked Mack what it was about the thought of being late that makes him anxious, and he was a bit flummoxed. Under closer interrogation though, he came up with a few plausible answers.

First, the worry of missing something. That struck me as odd, but I suppose my question was a bit vague – I hadn't specified what he was going to be late for. And I'm guessing he was thinking of something like a film, a lecture or group meeting – something that would start without him.

Next, the need to settle before going in. That makes a lot of sense and applies to a lot more situations. Almost all in fact.

Next again, being perceived as rude. I suppose if you don't have an excuse, this would look like rudeness. But if you're delayed for a good reason that a reasonable person would understand, I'd have hoped that would reduce the anxiety. I don't think it does for Mack though.

Finally, not being able to dictate how the room looks. Ah, he's thinking of business meetings again – especially adversarial ones. However, it could equally apply to meeting people in a café, bar or restaurant, because if you're last you could find yourself in the least sensory friendly position if all the other seats are already taken.

It was interesting to read through Autie blogs and find that this anxiety about being late is a common thing. Not so much the *being* late even; but the *fear* of it.

7 March

Last week, we arrived in good time for a medical appointment and sat for the obligatory 20 minutes in the car before Mack went in just a little ahead of time. Unfortunately, the person he was going to see was running 20 minutes late, by which time he was pretty agitated.

Normally, Mack takes it as rudeness or disrespect if someone's late – which explains one of his answers about why he so desperately needs to be early himself. But when it's a medical appointment, he worries that he's been forgotten. Or sometimes he starts catastrophising on behalf of whoever the medics are overrunning for, which makes him feel guilty for being there at all. Either way, he's now up to high doh which has undone all the mental preparation he'd gone through to be ready and settled for his appointment.

☉ **The need to be punctual (or early) is rooted in the need to be prepared, calm and in control.**

Mack is great at keeping me informed. If he's visiting the kids, for example, he'll call or send a text just as he's leaving and give me an ETA so that I know when to expect him home. Very thoughtful, isn't he? Except that he'll say he'll be home in about three-quarters of an hour but actually arrive only 20 minutes later. Clearly, it's something to do with this fear of being late or need to be early.

Every time it happens, I kick myself for being a slow learner. I should *know* by now to allow for his time warping – especially if I'm famished and want to have dinner ready for the moment he walks through the door.

> <<I know that it shouldn't really matter – Shonagh rarely gives me an ETA herself, after all. But if I don't let her know I'm on my way and then I crash, she won't know to start worrying and call for search and rescue! On the other hand, if I give a realistic time, I'll spend the whole journey worrying that I'll be late, which would probably increase my chances of crashing...>>
>
> Mack

☉ **Being early is simply another way of being prepared and in control. It's key to managing anxiety.**

Takeaways for Mack
- If something happens to make him late, remember that it doesn't actually matter – nothing bad will happen.

Takeaways for me
- Allow for his need to be early when making plans.

- Remember to proportionately adjust any ETAs he gives me so that, no matter what he says, I can set my own, more realistic expectations!

> <<I was on my way to visit one of the kids and there was a crash on the motorway. While *I* was fine, someone else clearly wasn't, and a huge tailback ensued which must have added about an hour onto my journey. I wasn't over-worried about this because, as usual, I'd allowed myself plenty time in case of exactly this kind of scenario. I'm pretty sure I made it roughly on time.
>
> However, what I hadn't appreciated was that the kids are so used to me doing the early thing that they were getting worried because I was 'late'! I was happily oblivious, strumming away to Bryan Adams, while they'd been busy sending each other and Shonagh panicked messages about what might have befallen me. Bit of an own goal there.>>
>
> Mack

Reluctantly, I have to admit there are some upsides to being early for everything. For example, Mack always argued that having time for a thorough recce before any kind of business pitch or meeting gave him an advantage over the competition. Outside of work, being first generally means getting the best seats, best bargains or best tickets. And, given airlines and hotels always overbook, arriving early means you're not the ones to get bumped!

Impulsiveness

8 March

Mack has always been impulsive. Take cars, for example. When he decides the time has come for a change, he researches options thoroughly and, once he's decided on the type he wants, he'll choose from what's available *right now*. I'll say to him, "But you hate a black interior, why not just keep an eye out till one with a light interior comes up?" But he can't wait.

The first time I changed my own car after Mack came into my life, I dragged him round several garages with me. Nothing I saw or tried particularly appealed, and by the time we'd been round three or four showrooms, he was looking a bit jaded. Until we hit the Mazda garage, that is, where I found myself drooling over a beautiful little red roadster – an MX5 – well over my budget.

Five minutes later, Mack came bounding over to me (I was still stroking the red roadster) to say he'd found one, right on budget, round the back. I was thrilled to bits – till he showed me it and my heart sank like a stone. "…It's black." I told him. "*Yes!*" he said as though that was the best thing ever. He clearly hadn't registered my tone or my expression. "No, it's *black*!" I repeated flatly, "And it's got those mean, slitty little eyes." "*Yes!*" he beamed again, as if that made it even better, "It's a Mark 1". He still didn't get it and was so busy purring over the mean machine that he remained oblivious to my complete antipathy towards it. He was all for doing a deal there and then. But there was no way I was going to buy a black car with mean, slitty eyes, so I bust the budget and bought the red Mark 2. I should have realised way back then that he was going to be a bad influence on me!

I've changed my car twice since then – I like to make them last – succumbing both times to Mack's impulsiveness. While I love my current car, the other one was a huge mistake. Smart, comfy and with all mod cons, it turned out to be a lawnmower and I regretted that purchase almost immediately. I could have *crawled* up a hill faster.

Mack buys houses in much the same way. However, I've discovered the trick is to view a whole bunch of properties on my own and then present him with an acceptable shortlist. Otherwise, who knows where we could end up!

And then there's shopping. While Mack hates going to high street or retail park stores – which are full of people, lights and noise – he seems to love buying things online. From my point of view, the only saving grace is the 14-day right to cancel and return. Otherwise, he'd probably be destitute by now. With online shopping, he gets the thrill of buying an item but, if and when remorse sets in, he can get his money back. So I don't worry too much about his clicking impulse.

The question is, is impulsiveness an Autie thing? Back to Google. The first hit returned was an Autie forum where someone had asked exactly the same question about her own husband. The answers all suggested a strong link between autism and impulsivity – which appears to be psychology terminology for impulsiveness.

😮 **Autism is often characterised by a lack of impulse control and autistic people tend not to give much thought to the consequences of their impulsivity.**

> <<I'm not impulsive: I'm *decisive*. And that's a good thing. This world needs people who can make decisions rather than prevaricate, procrastinate or vacillate. For people like me – for whom catastrophe lurks round every

corner – there's no time to waste, so why mess about?!>>

Mack

OK, I admit we're at opposite ends of the decisiveness scale, but I do like to think things through rather than beat myself up after making a hasty and poor decision. Like the lawnmower. And sometimes procrastinating *does* pay off. How many times do you receive an email from a boss or customer asking for something that's going to be difficult and laborious, only to receive another email a few days later saying they've changed their minds? Sorry, we've strayed off-piste again.

9 March

We were trying to ascertain the nature of the link between autism and impulsiveness – I mean, decisiveness. But it seems that the jury's out on this.

If impulsivity isn't a *symptom* of autism, could the link be a by-product of other Autie traits?

Uncertainty for example. We know Auties hate that, and anything that involves making a decision is surely all about ending uncertainty. So, wondering whether or not to move house? Mack needs an answer *now* – yes or no. What house to buy? "*That* one!" (often the first one viewed). How much to bid? Forget sealed bidding, he'll want to whack in an over-the-odds offer for acceptance by 5pm.

Another possible explanation is his need to finish. Mack finds activities that drag on excruciating, so deciding to move and then spending weeks viewing houses and debating over them is agony for him. If you could sell and buy online the very same day you decide to move, he would.

However, this isn't the only kind of impulsiveness Mack shows. He's generous by nature so he'll enthusiastically make all sorts of offers to people without thinking about the implications. For example, a tradesman will admire one of the boy toys or tools he's bought for his various renovation projects. The correct response is to agree that it's a great toy or tool – or rubbish it if it's not. However, Mack will either give it away or, if it was expensive, offer to sell it to them at a bargain price or barter it to knock the cost of a job down. He's thrilled with himself – as is the tradesman – but it's a scunner the next time we need that particular item for a job!

Similarly, he'll offer to help someone out if or when they seem to be struggling or procrastinating. His offer is sincere because he wants to help, but then he realises he's committed to something that's going to cause him sensory and social hell. I'm not sure what drives this kind of impulsivity, other than a lovely nature, but we're going to need to get a handle on it so that he doesn't keep overcommitting. As we now know, that road leads to overload, exhaustion and the stone wall.

> <<I used to do a little portrait photography outside of the day job and, if I say so myself, I was pretty good at it. So when Juliana mentioned that she and Roderick weren't going to engage a professional photographer for their wedding, I happily offered to take the photos.
>
> I'm not sure I'd completely thought it through though. I guess, at the time, I was thinking only of the upsides; it would be a lovely wedding gift, I enjoy taking and producing photos, and I find social occasions easier if I have a job to do. What I'd omitted to account

for – never mind the Autie-related trauma of the journey and staying in a party villa for a whole week – was what I now recognise as the combined effect of sensory overload and social anxiety. While the job I'd given myself meant I could hide behind a lens, I wouldn't be able to escape, even for the short respites that might ordinarily help me get through a social event.

I realised, shortly after making the offer, that I'd dug a hideous hole for myself. What if I had a meltdown on the day and couldn't do it?!

Luckily, Juliana mentioned that there would be at least a couple of others there who also fancied themselves as photographers. A potential lifeline! I quickly forged a cunning plan that would not only reduce the stress I'd heaped on myself, but provide a safety net… I handed out memory cards to the others and asked them to send me their best shots after the event so that I could make up an album for Juliana and Roderick using the best of the best we had between us.

Thankfully, the plan worked. My stress levels were reduced – albeit only slightly – the others were happy to send me their best photos and, not least, I was able to produce a great album from our combined efforts.>>

Mack

☺ **Decisiveness is great, but sometimes the speed of a decision can be at the expense of its quality.**

Takeaways for Mack
- Consider the consequences of any decisions he makes.
- Limit the downsides of an impulsive decision given our new understanding of the autistic mind.
- It's not just a lady's prerogative to change her mind – he can too!

Takeaways for me
- Keep applying the brakes when appropriate. And possible!

Compulsiveness

10 March

To the layman – me! – impulsive means the need to do something *right now*, and compulsive means the need to do something – the same thing – *again and again*.

Happily, Mack doesn't have this to any great degree. He certainly doesn't have OCD – I know that because I've googled it and I'm pretty sure we'd know all about it if he did. OCD takes you into the realms of excessive, obsessive and compulsive recurring thoughts and repetitive behaviours that you can't control, and it can seriously hamper your life. I mean, even more than certain aspects of autism have done.

We've already touched on some things that could be considered compulsions – the continual security checks, socket/switch checks and tidying up. But you could easily argue that Mack is simply a tidy and security-conscious person, and I'd need to concede that.

So why am I looking into this?

Well, there are a few other little things that Mack does time and time again that I'm struggling to explain, and I guess I'm just curious to know if this is part of being an Autie.

The most worrying is his inability to simply chill out while there's anything at all that he considers needs to be done or finished. And even when there isn't. Right now, he's knackered and, in my view, there's nothing that needs to be done today. But will he sit in the sunshine and just have a lazy afternoon? Not in this lifetime. *Why*?!

He tells me, "I feel guilty." That takes me back to my childhood, when I knew I should tidy my room but *so* didn't want to. I'd read, write, draw, anything but tidy my room – but as soon as I heard a foot on the staircase, I'd leap up and make as if I were tidying. But Mack's a grown-up now, with no one to answer to. So why doesn't he feel that he can simply do what he likes, when he likes, how he likes? He can't give a satisfactory answer to that other than he feels he ought to be doing something to justify his existence. It's his default setting.

The truth is, he's in a dark place just now and if he sits down with nothing to occupy his mind, the monsters creep up on him. I hope it won't always be this way, but I know he's going to continue to struggle for a while yet. And I'd rather he carried on pottering about than slip deeper and deeper into that black hole.

11 March

😲 **The compulsions of someone with OCD get in the way of activities they value. This is not the case for autistic people who may actually value a compulsion – to stim for example.**

As with impulsivity, could the link between compulsiveness and autism be a by-product of other Autie traits?

Mack's explanation that he ought to be doing something "to justify his existence" is telling. That goes right back to the lack of self-worth that's so very common among Auties due to childhood experiences of bullying, rejection and abuse.

The depression is undoubtedly another factor in Mack's need to keep himself occupied. And related to that is his catastrophising.

While keeping busy is his default at the best of times, he's worse when he's in full catastrophising mode. In the run up to his operation, he's been in overdrive, convinced he's going to die under the general anaesthetic. But he's not howling in a corner, full of woe; he's dealing with it by being practical and organised.

First, he updated his will and put a living will/advance directive in place too. Second came worries about me being left to manage everything by myself. "I don't want to leave you in a mess so I need to do all these jobs – you can't sell the bolthole with work needing done." And then there's his business. "I need to appoint you as a director so you can manage it and close it down."

This isn't the first time he's believed he was imminently about to meet his maker. Back in the day, I genuinely used to wake up of a morning and check he was still breathing. It was always a relief to find he was. While I hadn't done that in 15 years or so, I've done it again a few times in the run up to this op – his anxiety must be catching!

Among his cheerier compulsions are buying clothes and cars. I watched Chris Packham's *Asperger's and Me* a while back and was amused to see Chris's wardrobe[24]. Row upon row of identical or similar items of clothing. Mack does that too – he just doesn't file and display them as beautifully. But when he finds something he likes or that's a particularly good fit, he'll buy several – virtually all in black, grey or navy. To be fair, sometimes his shirts will have a little splash of colour in them, but nothing else has. When daughter Halle was with us during lockdown, she made him sell dozens of now out-of-fashion shirts, jumpers and jackets, many of which still had their tags on!

---

[24] Vimeo (2017), Chris Packham: Asperger's & Me. Accessed March 2023 at:
https://vimeo.com/252876361

Cars I've already mentioned. 29 in 22 years averages nine months per car. He doesn't actually turn them over as regularly as that though – when times were hard, he drove a clapped-out banger for a year or two and then a bottom-of-the-range leased car for a three-year period. When times were better, he ran a couple of cars at a time.

> <<What Shonagh's omitting to tell you is that there's generally been a very good reason to change a car.
>
> The one I had when I first met her, for example, I sold to fund the start-up of my business. I traded down and down again and then, after 9/11, I was broke and for the next couple of years had to drive a 12-year old banger that Dad had been allowing to rust in his back yard. For the next 15 years or so the cars I had were all leased through the company because I needed a reliable car to travel around the country from client to client for work.
>
> The reason I got through so many leased cars is that some of them were downright dangerous. I had a red Seat – the electrics failed on the motorway during a heavy downpour while my kids were in the back. I wasn't driving that again! I had a Skoda whose engine blew – they replaced it with one of a colour I couldn't abide. I had a Subaru Outback that I loved, but its clutch blew out. I had a Merc C class whose brakes failed.
>
> These problems continued even after I started owning my own cars again. I had a Merc GLE that broke down in the middle of Dundee last

year and they couldn't find anything wrong with it. Well, I obviously couldn't keep it after that – I'm still gutted about that one...>>

Mack

☹ C'est la vie.

Takeaways for Mack
- Guilt is a ghost he needs to exorcise – having reached the ripe old age of 63, he's earned the right to put his feet up and consign anything and everything he likes to the chuck-it bucket.

Takeaways for me
- Encourage any pottering about that occupies his mind and distracts him from black thoughts.
- But try not to let him bash on with unnecessary manual labour his ageing bones can't handle and that will lead to fatigue.

Coping with illness

Diagnosis

12 March

As Mack had managed to bluff his way through life for 63 years, you could argue that getting a formal diagnosis of autism was a little academic. Indeed, if we hadn't discovered the cancer, he might never have pursued it. But given the extent to which he's struggled since hitting his wall, we knew there was no way he could get through cancer treatment without support.

That support has taken many forms and has involved many wonderful people.

First, the doctor Mack initially consulted about his raised PSA levels. It was he who set the cogs in motion towards the cancer diagnosis and, realising that Mack was struggling with more than cancer worries, also referred him to Nicol, the psychiatric nurse attached to their practice.

Second, Nicol. On recognising the nature and magnitude of Mack's challenges, he wasted no time in referring him to the community mental health team who, because of a very long waiting list for autism assessment, immediately referred Mack on to Number 6. Nicol also offered to help Mack with his PTSD.

Third, the team at Number 6, specifically Tom, Garry and Laurent. Tom and Garry conducted the assessments over a six-week period, and after confirming the diagnosis, offered Mack the ongoing support of Number 6's services. This included the opportunity to take part in the late diagnosis group sessions led by Autie facilitator Laurent.

<<I wasn't very sure about joining these sessions at first, but the fact that they were happening online rather than in person certainly made it much easier. I could never have imagined how useful they'd be.

I'd spent a lifetime feeling like a cuckoo in a family of dunnocks. Suddenly, here was a nest of fellow cuckoos! They thought like I did, had very similar experiences and reacted to things the same way, too. I could talk to them without having to mask or explain myself – they just got it. They got me. And to be honest, that in itself was a bit life-changing. To know I'm not the only cuckoo in the entire world was even more helpful to me than learning the hows and whys of the Autie mind. It made me feel, spiritually at least, a little less isolated.>>

Mack

While learning about autism has been hugely enlightening – and will be invaluable in helping Mack get through his cancer treatment and recovery – the main driver behind going for the autism diagnosis was to have it on his medical records. Our hope is that any medic picking up Mack's file will see that he's autistic and immediately understand that he may react differently to things and/or need reasonable adjustments to their normal procedures.

The results so far have been pretty positive.

The first step in our cancer journey was the MRI back in August. As I mentioned when exploring medical anxiety, Mack was unable to go through with the scan at his first appointment because he was caught off guard when they tried to strap him down. Although this incident took place before Mack's autism diagnosis, he did explain that his anxiety was probably due to autism. They kindly described his panic attack as "the most dignified meltdown" they'd ever seen, and they were very understanding and supportive.

His second attempt at the MRI came a couple of weeks later. Much more confident this time – because he now knew exactly what to expect – Mack didn't mention autism to anyone. The downside of this was that when he refused the injection of a contrast dye – which he'd done last time too because his research told him this can increase your risk of Alzheimer's – the doctor on duty that day tried to insist. Despite getting a bit stressed out about it, Mack thankfully remained articulate enough to explain himself and they eventually accepted his decision. The good news was that he successfully got through the MRI. The bad news was that it showed a suspicious shadow.

The second step was the biopsy, which made the MRI seem like a walk in the park. He really shouldn't have read up on the risks of transrectal biopsies – in retrospect, I'm astonished he went through with it, but I know it wasn't easy. Fortunately, nurse consultant Carole fell for Mack's woe-begone puppy eyes and she couldn't have looked after him better if he'd been her very own dog. Trust is crucial for Mack, and he trusted Carole. She was confident, patient, reassuring and gentle. She explained exactly what she was going to do and how long each step would take, and she counted down the steps and seconds just like his dentist does. She also had someone hold his hand throughout, and promised she'd stop the moment he said he couldn't go on.

One week later, we were back for the diagnosis, and it was Carole who broke it to us. To be honest, I was expecting a benign result. And I think, despite his worries, Mack was too. But Carole, upbeat and positive, stressed that a Gleason score of 3+4 (stage 2 cancer) was better for Mack than 3+3 (stage 1) would have been, because 3+3 means a recommendation of active surveillance. In other words, never-ending worry. She understood that Mack wouldn't be able to cope with that very well. 3+4 on the other hand means do something. Choose a treatment. Stop the cancer in its tracks and get back to living life, because cancer caught at this stage is perfectly curable. My ears pricked up at "perfectly curable" and I was awash with relief!

I can't be certain what was going on in Mack's head though. You'd expect him to have been quietly anxious and perhaps, on hearing that it was cancer, to go into a passive-play-dead type of meltdown. Not a bit of it. He was performing as though he were up for an Oscar, dripping informed medical terms, anticipating Carole's thoughts and finishing her sentences as though he were enthusiastically chatting about a cure for the common cold.

>> <<I had to be strong for Shonagh, as she dissolved when Carole turned to ask her how *she* was feeling. However, it was probably the hardest masking performance of my entire life. In one ear I was hearing I could die, and in the other my tinnitus had shot up to warp factor 10 – despite having vaguely computed the word 'curable'. I felt physically sick. But knew I had to get through it for Shonagh.

>> The use of medical terms – and understanding them because of my research – meant I could cut short the discussions on my potential demise. I guess I was still trying to do my control thing by managing, as much as

> possible, an uncontrollable situation. Once my head allowed a little space, I could hear a wee voice screaming, "I want out of here". I was close to meltdown but managed to hold it together, just. Don't know how.>>
>
> Mack

Carole explained that as there were risks associated with any prostate cancer treatment, Mack needed to choose for himself between the recommended options – surgery to remove the whole gland, or radiotherapy to zap the tumour. To help with his decision, she arranged an appointment with the surgeon to discuss the prostatectomy, and another with a consultant clinical oncologist to discuss radiotherapy. In the meantime, and during the long recovery from the biopsy, we had some space to digest the news and read up on the options.

I initially thought radiotherapy would be the way to go, especially when Carole showed us an image of the machine and I realised that it was a non-invasive procedure. It appeared that you just had to lie fully clothed on the table under a space-age device while it magically and invisibly zapped your cancer. Game on. But when she explained Mack would have to be zapped on 20 consecutive working days, I realised it was a non-starter. Game off again.

Why? Because getting Mack to a hospital appointment is a serious undertaking. It's not like going to the supermarket where he can just pop in his earplugs if sensory or anxiety issues creep up on him. Nope. A hospital appointment for anything more than, say, an ingrowing toenail, requires pre-numbing by diazepam and a smattering of propranolol. He's only had to use this combination of meds on a few occasions – for dental procedures – but the consequences are pretty unpleasant.

<<The diazepam makes my brain foggy, which is a slightly scary feeling for someone who strongly feels the need to be alert and in control. It also gives me shocking heartburn. And the propranolol can trigger really bad dreams – nightmares sometimes. As the meds start to wear off, I ache all over because the diazepam is a muscle relaxant and my body doesn't understand relaxed. But worse is the day after, when a wave of depression and tiredness hits me like a truck. And then reverses over me a few times for good measure. It can take a full week to recover.>>

Mack

If that's what it's like taking the meds for *one* appointment, there's no way he could get through a course of radiotherapy – he'd stop taking them after a few days and then go into a full-blown meltdown. Not an option. It's bad enough doing a runner from the dentist's, it's altogether another to abscond from cancer treatment.

Mack's first reaction on hearing Carole confirm it was cancer, was an immediate, "Get it out!" That, of course, means surgery – for most people a more radical solution. And although that would be a one-and-done approach, it also entails a general anaesthetic and a long recovery.

Recovery is another matter and a relative term – it seems that no one escapes either of these treatments without their quality of life being impaired to some extent.

As a result of his tendency to catastrophise, Mack had a head start on me when it came to researching the options. I'd been so sure it would be benign that I hadn't investigated anything beyond the biopsy – but he'd already read up on the surgery, external beam radiotherapy, hormone therapy, brachytherapy, cryotherapy... and didn't much like the sound of any of them. And I have to admit that, on wading my way through all the literature myself, I felt much the same way.

At this point, I got in touch with my friend Brodie who had already faced this same dilemma himself a few years before. I clearly remembered him saying that he hadn't much fancied any of the options offered to him either, so had ended up going to London to have some experimental treatment done privately. He'd been more than happy with the outcome. I couldn't even remember what he'd called the procedure, but Brodie is nobody's fool, and I knew he would have researched it inside out before making his decision.

HIFU it was called, which means high intensity focused ultrasound. If I understand it correctly, you lie under another space-age device to get zapped, but by ultrasound in this case rather than radiotherapy. And it's a one-and-done zapping, not 20 days' worth. While Scotland still considers it to be experimental – because there's not enough *long*-term data available to compare it with the other treatments – they've been doing it in England for donkey's years. It's minimally invasive, you can be riding a bike again within days, and there are fewer risks. For many, like Brodie, it doesn't impair quality of life at all. It sounds like a no-brainer to me, but of course nothing's ever that simple.

The downsides from Mack's point of view are: "I'll probably not come round from the general anaesthetic." OK, that puts it on a par with the surgery – nothing lost, nothing gained. "By definition, it's only focusing on the existing tumour, but prostate cancer is multi-focal so I might get more tumours." True, but you can simply get the new tumours zapped if that happens, and your quality of life may not have been impaired in the meantime. "I'd have to go to London because they don't do it here – the travel, a whole week in a place I won't know or be comfortable." I admit, that would be stressful in his current head space. "The uncertainty of not knowing if it'll come back..." OK, that's a biggie. "And, it'll cost about 20 grand all in." The money is neither here nor there – we'd find it somehow – but I know it's not really the financing of it that's the problem. The truth is that the little voice that was screaming, "Get it out!" after the diagnosis, still is.

We created a spreadsheet to compare the risks of all the treatments, but it's really hard to get truly comparable figures. There are so many variables, and you can't drill down to any meaningful level of detail – though, truth be told, the details are a distraction anyway. The only real choice for *my* vintage Autie is between the surgery and the HIFU. Had HIFU been available here in Edinburgh, that might have swung it. Or maybe if Scotland was prepared to pay for it to be done on the NHS in England… But a reply from the Scottish Government confirmed that wouldn't be happening.

13 March

We received the diagnosis mid-September and the meetings with the oncologist, surgeon and HIFU man were all completed by mid-December. At which point Mack was officially added to the four-month waiting list for surgery. Yes, that little screamer has won the day.

Going through the diagnosis process and facing an illness like this would be hard for anyone, but for someone who is autistic, there are a few things that make it a little harder.

For Mack, the catastrophising is a big issue. As I mentioned before, he's updated his will, put an advance directive in place, made me a director of his business and thrown himself into every DIY job that might possibly need done to ready the bolthole for sale if he isn't going to be around. Disaster mitigation. Has it helped? Hard to say. I haven't seen a reduction in his anxiety levels, but it's given him a bit of focus which, for a while, makes him feel a little less helpless.

Not feeling in control is, to Mack, the monster under the bed. The researching helped. Again, it lent him some focus, and the fact that there was a choice of treatments – albeit equally unappealing ones – meant he had a measure of control over that, at least. No one was pushing him in any particular direction and he had time to decide which was the best option for him. No pressure. In theory.

While the primary reason for going with the surgical option is to remove rather than just zap the cancer, this doesn't *guarantee* he'll be cancer-free. We won't have certainty that it hasn't spread elsewhere until they've done the histology after the operation. And that uncertainty continues to worm its way around Mack's over-exercising Autie brain.

His anxiety levels have been stratospheric for the medical appointments, particularly the biopsy, increasing his dependence on meds. And for the last few weeks, he's needed propranolol almost every day. But the worst of the demons Mack has struggled with since the cancer first raised its ugly head is depression, which has hit him in waves.

> <<It took me a while to get my head around the diagnosis. I expect most people feel that though. "Why me?", "What have I done to deserve this?" Or, "I must be a horrible

person to deserve this". I can't believe anyone would take it in their stride. But maybe others find it easier to talk about the deep-rooted fears and sense of helplessness that come with a critical illness like cancer. I've often felt overwhelmed by it.

It was great to be able to speak to Brodie about his experience, and to his pal Chalky who had been through the surgery. It's easier to talk to people who have been where you are now – you don't have to struggle to explain yourself and you know they're in your corner. They were both very kind and supportive and helpful.

When I felt most like I was drowning, I called Prostate Cancer UK and spoke to their specialist nurses. Once to discuss specific worries about my treatment options and probable outcomes, and another time simply for a shoulder to cry on. That also helped a lot, and it's a relief to know they're there if and when I feel I'm going under.>>

Mack

Treatment

15 March

According to my investigations, autistic people experience more pain, anxiety and pain-related fear than neurotypical people[25]. This is presumed to be because of sensory differences and because Auties process pain in a different way. Essentially, they tend to have a lower pain threshold.

Mack definitely experiences more anxiety and pain-related fear, but I'm puzzled about his pain threshold. He'll yell, "Ow!" if I give him a static shock, or if I turn over in my sleep and inadvertently kick him. But while I barely notice either the shock or the collision, Mack reacts like a wounded puppy. And yet, if he's engrossed in a DIY activity and hurts himself, he often doesn't notice until later when he's surprised to find he's bleeding or bruised. I know I'd want a lot more sympathy if it had been *my* hand jammed in the car door the other week – his blackened nail is still hanging in there! – but he's always sporting an array of wounds so perhaps he's just hardened to a certain level of discomfort.

I can't find a clear explanation for why Mack would find some things more painful and others less. So I've decided it must be because pain perception is dulled if an Autie is absorbed in something. That would seem to fit with the finding that Auties with poor proprioception can still show incredible dexterity when concentrating – if you're engrossed, you're using up all your brain power on the job in hand and have no bandwidth left for acknowledging pain.

---

[25] Failla MD, Gerdes MB, Williams ZJ, Moore DJ, Cascio CJ (2020), Increased pain sensitivity and pain-related anxiety in individuals with autism. Pain Rep. 2020 Nov 16;5(6):e861. doi: 10.1097/PR9.0000000000000861. PMID: 33235944; PMCID: PMC7676593.

Unless you've drilled through your foot or hacked a few digits off, of course. Again, just a theory.

Pain perception aside, we need to manage Mack's anxiety and pain-related fear as best we can to get him through the treatment. So it was probably a good thing that we faced quite a long wait from making the treatment decision in mid-December to the next step, which was the pre-op meeting yesterday. The worry never really receded, but the time-lag did give Mack some space to get his head round the *autism* diagnosis and understand his own reactions to the challenges involved in facing scary illness.

That understanding helped us prepare for the pre-op meeting. As you'd expect, Mack had done masses of homework beforehand so that he had a good idea of what would be happening. As usual before a stressful medical appointment, he took a little diazepam the night before to ensure he'd get some sleep. And, topping up next morning, we set off with silly time to spare just in case of any delays en route and so that he'd have time to settle himself before we went in. To kill the hour spent in the car park, we munched our way through a lavish picnic lunch of ham sandwiches and coke – living the high life, as ever! – and set out 15 minutes early with his emergency kit and our folder full of notes and questions.

First, we met with a lady called Lorna. When Mack introduced himself, he handed her his autism card – the first time it he'd ever used it – and all credit to her, Lorna took it in her stride. She was amazing in fact. As though she dealt with Auties every day.

She began by taking blood pressure readings but, noting they were sky high, decided to come back to that later in the hope that they'd drop during the appointment. Next, she rattled through all the questions she needed to ask – but took time to elicit any additional details about his relevant health, allergy, fitness and medication history. Then, she asked about any questions or worries we might have. By that stage however, she'd already covered pretty much everything we'd wanted to ask, other than concerns specifically relating to Mack's autism.

Thanks to Number 6 and our investigations, we were able to explain to Lorna easily and succinctly the impact of Mack's autism on his ability to cope with hospitalisation. She was great about it. In addition to the usual blurb she must have to go through with all patients, she talked us through what to expect from arrival to discharge. She also offered to bend normal procedures to allow me to stay with Mack for as long as possible before the surgery. And while she couldn't promise that a side room would be available, she could promise there would be no more than four people to a room. What's more, they'd put him in a corner facing the door, and make sure any aids he might need – such as earplugs – would be to hand should he begin to have any sensory or anxiety issues on coming round.

Then it was back to the tests – bloods, oxygen, ECG and blood pressure. The blood pressure looked to be the only concern – it was still up at 168/92 despite the meds – but I'm sure they'll figure out how best to deal with that.

By the end of that appointment, Mack was still upright but definitely looking in need of a sugar boost, so our next stop was the hospital café. And then on to his next appointment which was with a physio and nurse specialist Alexander. That was a harder meeting because it brought home the reality of what was happening and how hard Mack will have to work in an attempt to limit the impact of the prostatectomy on his quality of life. Depressing stuff, but you wouldn't know it if you'd been a fly on the wall. Comic banter, innuendo, uproarious laughter – it was like watching an episode of *Live at the Apollo*, with Mack in full performance mode.

23 March

The fallout from the effort of attending these meetings wiped the next week from Mack's calendar. Exhaustion first – it set in within half an hour of leaving the hospital – followed by the black cloud of depression – at its very worst the next day – followed by physical pains and palpitations as the meds wore off. There are no Autie tricks we've discovered to help with this, but at least we now understand why it happens and know to write those days off.

The day after the pre-op meeting, we were given a date for the surgery. Sadly, it was to be at a different hospital – St John's in Livingston rather than the Western General in Edinburgh – which turned our expectations upside down and added an extra layer of anxiety to the mix. We would now need to plan for at least one trip to scope out the journey, the parking, the building and the unit or ward at St John's. We were also worried that some of the assurances Lorna gave us may no longer apply.

This week, however, Mack received another call, this time from a lady at St John's. Amazingly, it felt as though she – Marsali – had been a fly on the wall at our previous meetings and conversations, as she had a complete understanding of Mack's 'need to know' and the concerns we'd raised about being able to cope on the day. It's hard to know who to thank for this exceptional communication – we hadn't expected the service to be so well joined up and it was a huge relief.

Marsali offered to meet with us two weeks before the surgery so that we could do a recce and Mack could meet key people he'd likely see on the day. It sounds like a little thing, but it meant a lot.

>><<I was astonished at quite how much the pre-op meetings took out of me. I'd felt absolutely hellish for a full week afterwards, and that was despite the fact that I was already familiar with the environment and had known roughly what to expect. God alone knows how hard I'll find the day of the surgery in any case, never mind it happening in a hospital I've never been to before and where everything and everyone will be unfamiliar. So when Marsali offered to meet with us, I was glad to accept.

> In the context of having a bit of your insides taken out, it probably sounds like a small thing. And I guess it is. But removing uncertainties to do with the environment could reduce my anxiety levels from 100 to, who knows, 95. And every little helps!>>

> Mack

5 April

We knew that Mack would be asked to report for surgery at either 7am or 11am; what we didn't know was whether we could request the 11am option or indeed whether it would make a difference or not. But as it turned out, we'd only just parked up for our recce appointment when Mack got a call to confirm it would be 11am. Phew. That's great news for me, because I'm *so* not a morning person. But it will also mean that Mack has much more time to settle. I think. Perhaps they reckoned that too.

The recce was well worthwhile. Now we know exactly how long to allow for the journey – because the appointment with Marsali was taking place at exactly the same time on exactly the same day of the week – as well as how long to allow for the inevitable cut-throat hunt-the-parking-space challenge. A stressful experience in itself. You could almost *see* Mack's blood pressure begin to rise at this point.

A few minutes later, we arrived at the main entrance, still in good time. However, it was pretty busy inside and the echo of hubbub and hustle'n bustle bounced off the walls all around us. And suddenly I found myself alone in the mêlée, wondering momentarily if Mack had done a runner. It wouldn't be the first time. I once had to attend a dental appointment in his stead – while he darted back to the refuge of the car – so that we didn't completely waste the poor dentist's time. Again. Just as well I'd needed a filling anyway.

Thankfully, he'd just taken a moment to regroup in the gents, and soon we were following the red line, as directed, to the day surgery unit to meet Marsali. Getting lost only once on the way!

Marsali was lovely, but boy was she a whirlwind. I guess you have to be, given the pressures the NHS is under. Anyway, she kindly gave us a lightning tour, showing us where we would check in on the day, where we would be taken for Mack to settle in and have his checks and chats, and where the theatres were. She showed us one of their three identical side rooms – the one they'll give Mack assuming he's not trumped by a medical emergency – as well as walking us through the whole ward so that Mack could identify alternative beds he'd feel comfortable with if it turns out he can't get a side room. As the beds were all in bays of four, this wasn't too daunting a thought – so long as he can be in a corner, protected from as much sensory stimulation as possible.

As Lorna had done, Marsali assured me that I could stay with Mack right up until he was due to be taken in for his surgery. What's more, she introduced us to her deputy, Rochelle, who would be on duty on the day and who kindly took a few minutes to chat with us and establish a wee rapport with Mack. Marsali would be back on duty the day after the surgery and promised to see him again then.

And that was it – done and dusted within 15 minutes! While my head was spinning with the speed and efficiency of it all, Mack had clearly had enough, so the timing was probably ideal as far as he was concerned. But rather than rush straight back to the car, he was keen to stop by the café for a sugar boost and a decaf coffee to go.

Even after all we've learned about autism, I still automatically take his behaviour at face value and think, "Oh, he must be feeling OK, then." Numpty me. Turns out he desperately needed a coffee to warm up his virtually frost-bitten hands, all the blood having deserted them in favour of heart-pumping in readiness for fight or flight. But he was also still in deep mask mode – forcing himself to stay calm while in a public place – and was convinced that making himself stop and interact in the café would be a useful desensitising exercise. Don't they call that self-flagellation?

> <<The habit of masking, coping, performing – whatever you like to call it – is so engrained I can't seem to stop. Shonagh continually reminds me, "You don't have to do this" and tells me to give myself a break. But I think that would be disastrous.

While I admit I'd been finding life tougher in the few years running up to the Covid pandemic, lockdowns and restrictions during 2020 and 2021 really put the kybosh on my ability to function socially, to engage and interact with others. Many of what I now recognise as Autie symptoms became worse when I was no longer having to mix with people every day – professionally or socially – and I guess I must have fallen out of the habit.

So, while the rest of the world has long since reverted to 'old normal', I still feel like I'm in some kind of internal lockdown. I *have* to find a way to turn this around. One café at a time, perhaps.>>

Mack

6 April

As the surgery date gets closer, Mack's capacity to cope with even routine demands on his psyche shrinks ever further. Nipping over to his sister's for lunch, for example, or having someone pop in for coffee. These are things he would have been able to plan for and cope with quite easily not so long ago – and hopefully will again once he's recovered. But for now? Not so much.

To help me get my head round this, I try to think of instances in my own life when I've felt that way. The only one that pops to mind goes back decades, when a work bully (my direct supervisor) was making my life hell. As well as bad-mouthing me to everyone, she set a number of traps – directing me to do things that I couldn't at that time know were wrong – in an attempt, I imagine, to get me into trouble or even sacked. At least one of which I fell headlong into!

The stress was all-consuming, and the only way I could cope was by keeping alert to the dangers and thinking of pretty much nothing else night and day for those few weeks. Because if I allowed myself to be distracted, the stress and dread would return like a tidal wave when I came back to earth – better to remain battle-hardened throughout than relax between assaults, I thought. I'm not sure if that's quite how Mack feels, but I can certainly relate to not having the mental space for fluffy stuff when something crushing is looming over you.

So, any remaining 'fluff' between the recce meeting and the day of the surgery has been removed from the calendar, and out have come all the letters, leaflets and research findings pertaining to the prostatectomy. We need to keep the beast in sight and make sure we're fully prepared to meet it!

First up is making sure Mack is fit for the surgery – which we've been doing for a while – following all the advice on how to reduce the risk of complications and improve his rate of recovery. To be fair, Mack was already in pretty good shape for a 63-year-old. His daily step count is generally between 10,000 and 20,000 due to agitation alone, so he hasn't felt the need to get on the treadmill. And for several months, he's been doing weird pelvic exercises to strengthen the muscles around and about the bit they'll be chopping out.

Nutrition is another important factor. Despite the many things Mack can't eat, we generally have a pretty good diet – not counting my proclivity for chocolate, of course. However, Lorna did advise us to increase Mack's intake of carbs in the run up to the surgery. Potatoes, rice, pasta, bread. I'm not sure it's made much difference to Mack, but it's certainly meant I've piled on the pounds – I'll be able to donate blood soon!

In the fortnight before the surgery, Mack was to stop taking any vitamins – such as D or B12 – or drinking alcohol. That was a bit of a blow because these are things that usually contribute to his wellbeing. When Mack's B12 levels drop, he's very susceptible to depression, and the occasional small glass of red wine at dinner time normally reduces his tension levels. And reduces blood pressure a little. Instead, he's had to rely more on his SAD lamp and meditation – with somewhat mixed success.

However, we're now about as prepared as it's possible to be. The last – and biggest – hurdle will be actually getting him to the hospital and keeping him there until they put him under. Several times he's been on the point of phoning to call it all off!

Probably the only thing that's kept Mack sane in the last two or three weeks is his bolthole outhouse project – a great distractor in itself as well as an opportunity for some man time with good pal Struie the joiner.

12 April

Mack has always had a tendency to perseverate and catastrophise and, since his autism diagnosis, I now understand why. Dealing with it can be tricky though. If he's perseverating about boys' toys or pastimes (the car, the outhouse/man cave, DIYing…), I've found it works well to fix an interested expression on my face while paying no attention whatsoever. However, there's always a danger that he might go seriously off on one – "I'm going to scrap that bloody car/demolish the conservatory/trash this kitchen" – so I daren't switch off completely!

Sometimes, he may be perseverating about something serious, and then it's important not only to listen, but to engage. For example, when he's ruminating about the cancer. And I'm still learning the ins and outs of this.

What I *do* know is that giving empty reassurances doesn't work – saying 'It'll be OK' to someone facing uncertainty is as helpful as saying 'Relax' to someone who's stressed out. It *is* reassurance Mack's looking for, I'm sure, but of a more constructive type.

Here's what I think's happening. A word of comfort or reassurance, while well meant, feels to Mack as though you're dismissing him, not taking his worries seriously. Rather than helping him to move on, it distresses him and is likely to prod him into repeating, elaborating, embellishing or exaggerating to convey how upset or anxious he is. It's a cry for help. But when *you* say, "It'll be fine," *Mack* hears, "I don't care". And if, despite his attempts to reach you, you continue to show you don't care, he'll feel abandoned, desolate, isolated, as if he's worthless and doesn't matter – all of which lead to the dark place.

I wish I knew how to really help. But the best I can do is listen and take his concerns on board – even if I don't share them (I *am* sure he'll be fine with the general anaesthetic!). What I've found is that letting him vent this way helps him to unload and usually, once he's done this, I find *he's* the one then doing the reassuring!

I came across an Autie forum the other day that touched on this, and they were talking about the difference between reassurance and validation. They were agreeing that 'It'll be OK' is more dismissive than helpful. Their preferred approach was for someone to acknowledge their worries and why they might feel the way they do – validation – and then go on to offer an alternative perspective. I get that and think that's what I'd prefer too. I hope this means I'm doing the right thing, but I still wish I had some proper counselling knowhow.

20 April

Finally, the big day arrived – 18 April. I think we'd both been expecting at least one major meltdown in those last few days, but it didn't happen. All our focus was on being organised and prepared for what Mack was now seeing as 'the inevitable'. We even had a timetable. 6.30am breakfast – the permitted cup of black tea and a slice of toast before fasting from 7am. 7am get showered and dressed. 8am double check overnight bag, emergency kit, paperwork, water and medication. 9am diazepam. 10am first 'pre-op drink', propranolol if necessary, water and leave for hospital. 10.15am second 'pre-op drink', finish water. 10.30am stop drinking anything. 11am check in… And yes, it went that smoothly – by 10.40am he was safely through the hospital doors, for real! Still no runner, still no meltdown.

Mack paid a quick visit to the gents while I waited for the receptionist at the ops admission desk to finish a call with another patient also due to check in at 11am – but who was stuck on the M8 because of a serious accident. In fact, three patients were held up in that same jam. I couldn't help but breathe a sigh of relief for Mack's anxiety levels that we'd been early and coming from the other direction.

But I was disappointed to learn that they weren't giving Mack a side room – they were all allocated 'for reasons of infection control'. In fact, Mack was OK with being in the bay initially (they put him in a lovely south-facing corner with an open window and a view!), but that night was a nightmare for him and it was a bit tough for his fellow patients when he had the inevitable panic attack at 3am. More on that later.

Student nurse Aggie settled Mack into his bay and, as promised, I was allowed to stay with him. There followed completion of the usual barrage of questions and pre-checks, including taking blood – which sadly took a few attempts through no fault of Mack's – and then the meetings with the anaesthetist and the surgeon, Arran.

Mack remained very calm and articulate throughout, and the only hint he gave that anything was wrong was when he said to me after Arran had left, "It's way too much, there's just so much information…too much to take in…". Actually, they were all saying exactly the same thing, and none of it was new, it was just that Mack's brain was beginning to freeze over – a meltdown of the passive-play-dead variety as happened at the airport in Spain all those years ago. Clearly, no one else could tell. Which reminded me; I'd forgotten to give them the note I'd prepared about his autism and how to manage his sensory sensitivity and anxiety – a suggestion I'd picked up from Autie articles online:

"Mack has been diagnosed as autistic. He suffers from:

- **Sensory sensitivity**. To minimise this, he's best in a side room failing which a quiet corner facing any noise and activity, with a clear escape route. He has ear plugs, music and an eye mask with him which may help.
- **PTSD**. Approaching or surprising him from behind can result in a panic attack.
- **High anxiety**. This is exacerbated by a hospital environment, needles, and a fear of the unknown. Needs to know exactly what will happen and when. Surprises result in panic attacks with sky-high blood pressure and heart rate. Uses propranolol on an as-needs basis to bring back down.

- **Dehydration and cramps**. Mack has no thirst reflex and, unless he's constantly reminded, he doesn't drink enough. Dehydration results in severe and painful cramping in his left calf, causing him to leap out of bed and bounce around.
- **Medication sensitivity**."

I quickly gave the note to Rochelle because, although they knew he was autistic, they were unlikely to understand much about what this meant for him and how best to handle any panic attack he might have.

Right on schedule, just about 1pm, robotic coordinator Lydia came to collect Mack and walk him to theatre. I felt a bit bereft as my zombie Autie dutifully wandered off with her, without a backward glance. Head bowed and shuffling along in his dressing gown and slippers, he reminded me a bit of the honey monster… Anyway, I have to say I hoped very much that he was wrong about the general anaesthetic – I didn't want that forlorn amble to be my last memory of my poor misunderstood husband.

> <<I was glad it was Lydia who came to meet me and walk me into surgery. I'd spoken to her on the phone a few times before so felt a little as though I knew her already. But in real life she was everything you'd hope she'd be. Friendly, good-humoured, relaxed and easy to chat to, but very much on the ball too. Her presence made me feel I was in good hands.
>
> On entering the theatre however, I was suddenly surrounded by a flurry of people who all seemed to want to touch me. The ground beneath my feet felt like quicksand – my ability to communicate was

disintegrating, and I could feel myself descending further into shutdown.

Happily, the anaesthetist took control – a pragmatic chap whom I'd met earlier. He didn't do much in the way of eye contact, and my first thought had been to wonder whether he was an Autie himself, but perhaps he was simply being considerate because he knew I was. Either way, he knew his stuff and instilled some confidence in me as he'd been very happy to take recognition of my worries and work round them. For example, my need to be aware of what was going on, my fear of sensory deprivation, and my preference for nasal prongs rather than a mask. Understanding my anxieties, he let me keep my glasses on and very quickly put me off to sleep!

I was expecting that to be that of course. My meet-your-maker moment. So I was as surprised as I was confused to wake up three hours later – glasses on – in the recovery room. *Alive.*>>

Mack

Recovery

21 April

The hospital staff were all lovely people, and all very good at their jobs. But I'm not sure they 'got' the whole autism thing. And I suppose that's not surprising as Mack had been performing as well as ever with everyone on the morning of the surgery. More subdued than normal to be honest, but no one would realise that if they hadn't met him before – he came over as being every bit as neurotypical as anyone else. So it was tricky to persuade them to let me see him again before visiting hour started at 7pm.

By 5.15pm, I'd asked three different people if I could get in to see him – all of whom disappeared never to be seen again – before accosting a nurse called Elaine who had popped into the discharge room where I was waiting. "Nope," she told me before I'd finished explaining why I wanted to see him, "not before 7." "But he's autistic…" I tried desperately, "Really?!" Elaine said, "I had no idea! Leave it with me…" And, star that she was, she got me in. Only for 10 minutes, mind you, and then I had to go back to the discharge room and wait till 7pm, but at least my mind was at rest. He really *wasn't* the one-in-100,000 who didn't make it through the general anaesthetic.

To be fair, Mack was so wabbit and groggy that I'm not sure it made any difference, my being there at that point. He was too exhausted to think straight never mind speak. So I left when visiting hour was over, promising to be back sharpish in the morning.

Unsurprisingly, it was a rough night for him, topped off at about 3am with a panic attack when his propranolol and surgical meds had worn off and he started to suffer the effects of sensory assault. The downside of being on an open ward. Snoring, rasping, coughing, ticking, humming, whirring, nurses quietly chatting and going about their duties such as doing obs and responding to call bells... Worse still, at one stage someone closed Mack's curtain fully, which meant he could no longer see the clock – the one thing that was keeping him sane as he counted down the minutes till morning and escape.

I had of course left them the note on what to do if this happened – give him some more propranolol, basically. But here's where the plan came unstuck.

Among the information the Western had given us was a green bag with an instruction to place Mack's meds in it on attending the hospital. We'd duly taken it along to St John's, only to be told they didn't do that there, so the green bag – with the propranolol – had gone back home with me. No matter, there was some in his emergency kit which was in his overnight bag. Mack *did* tell them this, but it seems they couldn't find it – presumably because of the subdued night-time lighting and the fact they were trying to be quiet so they didn't disturb too many other patients. Or maybe Mack just wasn't at his most articulate at that point. Thankfully, a very understanding nurse called Nuala scoured the hospital from top to bottom till she tracked down someone willing to donate a little propranolol, and then sat chatting with Mack for half an hour till he managed to settle again. For Mack, that night felt like never-ending purgatory but, thanks to Nuala, a strong sweet tea and his meditation app, he finally made it through till morning. The dawn chorus had probably never been so welcome!

Shortly after the chorus, the gents were encouraged to get up and start walking around again. However, while the others seemed to manage just fine, Mack found himself still very off-balance. Icky and woozy, he clung to the window sill to steady himself, trying to fend off looming panic.

<<Even with anti-sickness pills, the wooziness remained. In fact, I still feel a little as though I'm wearing anti-gravity boots after having popped some recreational drugs.

I wonder whether it's because I was in the Trendelenburg position for so long – that's the position they put you in for this operation, the table steeply tilted with your head towards the floor. It allows the surgeon greater access to pelvic organs. However, there are various side effects and I'm wondering whether this is one of them – exacerbated in my case because vestibular sensitivity is an aspect of my autism.

As with most things autism, more research is needed. But I'd certainly like to warn other autistics who are considering having an operation like this to be aware that it might happen to them too. Having said that, even though it's unpleasant it's still way better than the alternative!>>

Mack

Although Mack wasn't due to be discharged till the top of the day, I was back at the hospital by 9.30am. Bearing in mind how he'd run out of bandwidth before the op, I was desperate to be with him when they ran through the discharge information in case he was in a similar state. That would be a disaster. He'd mask beautifully, and then get home and have no idea what to do with the meds and catheter.

Turns out we were *both* a bit daunted by the debriefing!

First, Rochelle explained how to look after the catheter, which Mack would have to wear for the next couple of weeks, and what to do with the night attachments. Second, she talked about showering and looking after the six gruesome stab wounds across his tummy. Third, she ran through all the meds he'd have to take and when to take them – three different types of pill for the pain, some laxatives to get his system running again and, worst of all, blood thinning injections which, along with the Nora Battys (aka compression socks), would help prevent clotting. Yes, *do-it-yourself injections*! This came as a bit of a shock – and a blow given we're both needle-squeamish. And then there was all the what-happens-next stuff; appointments for a cystogram, removal of the catheter, another PSA test, the histology result...

It all seemed to make sense at the time, but you know what it's like. It's not till you get home that you realise you haven't retained it all or asked enough questions. What/how much are you supposed to eat? When are you allowed your first shower? How long do the dressings stay on for? Where exactly are you supposed to inject this stuff? What on earth is a cystogram?

An Autie on overload, Mack had retained even less than me – and poor Rochelle would have had no idea that half of it was washing over him, as he was masking as convincingly as ever. Thank God for Google. And, to be fair, we did have access to two former nurses, Halle and Marnie, so we at least had our 'phone a friend' to fall back on.

23 April

These first few days after the op have been full of anxiety-inducing milestones – the first injection, the first catheter night-bag, the first shower and change of dressings, the first poo!

The first injection was the one I'd been dreading most as I don't think I'd be any happier *giving* an injection than I am receiving one. But know what? I never got to find out. Although Mack feels exactly the same way about needles, his Autie control-freakery won out – he found he'd rather jab himself than relinquish control to another equally needle-phobic novice. It wasn't plain sailing though, "Oh God, is it supposed to hurt this much?!", "I must have done it wrong!", "What happens if I've hit the muscle or vein?!" Talk about stress-fest.

The catheter night-bag turned out to be fairly easy to attach, and once we were convinced it was working, we just had to learn to manage getting through the nights with it. This was a problem only because Mack would sleep for a couple of hours and then have to get up because of the pain. His big worry was that he might tread on the extended tube and accidentally rip the catheter out, so I'd have to move the bag out of the way while he manoeuvred out of the bed, and then he'd carefully dodge around it while shimmying to ease the discomfort and chaffing. It put me in mind of parties of yesteryear and women dancing round their handbags. Do people still do that, I wonder.

An even bigger dread for Mack was the changing of the dressings as he hadn't actually seen his wounds before. It made him feel a bit woozy and he had to lie down afterwards, but we got through that too.

I don't think you need to hear about the first poo – suffice to say it was a moment of joyous celebration.

26 April

One thing we hadn't really thought much about was medication sensitivity *following* the surgery. While the first few days of taking the meds went well, we were a bit paranoid about the risk of infection so were being hypercareful – we didn't want Mack to end up on antibiotics or have the catheter in for longer than necessary. But then strange things started to happen.

First was blood in the poo. A quick call with a doctor at his GP practice confirmed Mack should stop taking the ibuprofen, but that he needn't worry about the blood at this stage.

Then, on about the fourth night, he started to get 'jumpy' legs. I recognised immediately what he was describing – an inexorable achy-twitchy itch inside your legs that makes sleeping impossible. I suffered that for a couple of years – rarely nodding off before 3am because of it – until I realised it was a menopausal symptom and crushed it with patches. Turns out this is a rare but known side effect of the injections that he would simply have to endure until the course was over. Jumpy legs and a lack of sleep were preferable to a blood clot; a conclusion Mack could only agree with.

The doctor was also kind enough to flag another medication issue we'll need to consider. Looking ahead to the removal of the catheter, there's a possibility that if Mack fails the voiding test – which means if he can't pee without the catheter – it may need to be put back in. This normally involves the use of lidocaine, a local anaesthetic, but Mack won't be able to have this if he's using propranolol as the two drugs adversely react with one another. Typical. But a worry for another day…

And then he started reacting to the adhesive on the wound dressings – the skin around his sore tummy became screamingly itchy and needed a steroid cream.

It has to be said, Mack's GP practice have been amazing. While the rest of us have been struggling to get appointments for years – "You are now 10th in the queue", "No advance bookings available", "No appointments today, call again tomorrow" – Mack's surgery not only seem to take appointments and call back, but even make proactive calls.

A couple of months back, Mack developed shingles again. Because he was panicking about the impact this might have on his cancer appointments, as soon as he realised it might be shingles he called a phone doctor service and had it confirmed on video. This was just before 5pm one day. 9am next morning a doctor from his own practice called him – having received a report from the phone doctor service for his medical file – to ask how Mack was and if he needed anything. How terrific is that?!

The speed at which they'd managed to get him referred for the autism diagnosis was also incredible given the length of waiting lists for mental health support services. They'd clearly recognised that he was burnt out, and how important it would be to get the diagnosis on his file if he was going to have to face cancer treatment. Goodness only knows how Mack would have fared otherwise.

And they've been amazing since the op too. Despite the pressures GPs must be under, they've all taken the time to chat, to reassure and to help, quickly and responsively. Mack may not be the luckiest man alive, but he's certainly won the postcode lottery for GP services!

28 April

Despite the hurdles and the pains, Mack's mental health took a step change for the better as soon as the surgery was over. A dead weight had clearly been lifted. That's not to say he's been 'up' all the time – when he crashes, he crashes in style – but he has an underlying positivity that's been missing for a long while.

> <<It's a completely different kind of tiredness now. Yes, I'm exhausted, but it's lack of sleep and my body desperately needing rest to recuperate from its recent butchery; it's not the same crushing fatigue that had been plaguing me for so long before that.
>
> I know they say that I shouldn't have felt any symptoms of the cancer, but I'm not so sure. They're discovering more and more about autism and sensory sensitivity all the time, but unless that's your field of speciality, you're not going to know about it, are you?
>
> I'm sure it was the cancer, and now – I hope to God – it's gone!>>
>
> Mack

I've no idea whether there's something in that or not. It's possible, I guess. But he does have a lot of crazy theories, so who knows. Perhaps it's just the enormous dread of the last year or so having finally been lifted now that the surgery's behind us.

While some aspects of Mack's autism have made his cancer journey hard-going, others have been a great help. Researching, for example. You might think all he was doing was winding himself up by constantly feeding his need to know, but in fact it allowed him to prepare in ways that are making his recovery experience much easier than it might have been.

Here are just a few examples:

- The intubation from the surgery leaves you with a sore throat and dry cough. While the nurses taught Mack that pressing a cushion to his tummy during a cough would save him bursting his wounds – a truly invaluable tip! – his research suggested he invest in a breathing device. This has vastly reduced his coughing.
- Chatting to Brodie's friend Chalky – who had the same op done by the same surgeon several years before – was very helpful. Chalky's heartfelt advice was not to eat afterwards. He'd made that mistake, but his system couldn't cope – he threw up whatever they'd given him and ruptured his oesophagus, resulting in a significantly extended hospital stay. Mack's research showed that Chalky's experience of being unable to cope with food straight after surgery wasn't that unusual, so he knew to take only a little over the first day or two as his system rebalanced.
- When you leave hospital, the catheter is strapped to your leg just above and just below the knee. That's a lot of loose tubing just begging to get caught and accidentally ripped out. Mack came across a recommendation on an American site to secure it to the top of the leg to prevent the pulling. He duly invested in and attached an extra catheter strap when he got home and immediately felt the relief of the additional security. It hadn't been a pleasant experience to feel the catching and tugging of the tube before that!
- The catheter bag is bulky and needs constant access. While many sites suggest wearing 'loose clothing', one in particular recommended the type of joggers that have

a leg zip for returning home, and shorts for the rest of the time. Mack was more than happy to have followed this advice as it's made his catheter experience very much easier.
- You're advised to do the weird pelvic squeezes I mentioned earlier – Kegel exercises – in the run up to surgery and again after the catheter's removed to improve the chances – and rate – of recovering functionality down there. Mack found an app that both reminds him to do the exercises and times them, which he's found to be a great help.
- He also knew to stock up on items such as gels, surgical wipes, waterproof under sheets, and briefs rather than boxers, none of which we'd have had in the house otherwise.

There's only one thing we weren't properly prepared for, and that was seating. We'd identified chairs at home that we thought would be perfectly comfortable for Mack during his convalescence, but they turned out not to be. However, within 10 minutes of realising this, Mack had found a local supplier of mobility devices that had hospital chairs for hire, and so I had one in situ within the hour!

> <<I'm not sure there's anything online relating to prostate cancer that I haven't read – from medical articles and research findings to general information or advice and personal experiences. Some things were more helpful than others.
>
> The personal experiences of prostate cancer survivors were particularly useful – especially those written by positive people who were selflessly sharing in order to help others in the same situation. I didn't want to be exposed to

stories about the bleak emotional side of things – I was looking for factual information on how to mitigate the negatives as much as possible.

There was one American chap in particular who had done a series of videos charting his cancer experience as he went through it. It was matter-of-fact and honest but at the same time upbeat. He went into all sorts of details about what to expect at every stage of the journey, and I've found it exceptionally helpful.[26]>>

Mack

29 April

Within a few days of the surgery we were given an appointment for a cystogram, but there was no explanation of what this involved so I called to ask for more information. Basically, it was just an x-ray. If the results were fine, you were then sent to get the catheter out – which would entail hours of hanging around while drinking gallons of water for the voiding (peeing) test. Hmm. That didn't sound very Autie friendly to me.

Luckily, a lovely lady from the nurse urology unit called back to suggest a better plan. Attend the cystogram as per the appointment letter, but because it would be going like a fair at the urology unit that day, come back the *next* day instead to get the catheter out – that way, Mack would only

---

[26] YouTube (2015-2023), Mark's Prostate Cancer Experience. Accessed October 2022 to April 2023 at:
http://www.youtube.com/@prostatecancerexperience

have five other patients to contend with rather than 30. The NHS at their bendy best for us yet again.

> <<It's been the funniest thing, watching Shonagh stepping in to bat for me – I've never had anyone advocating for me before. I've always had to fight my own corner or, when I was little, hide in it – indeed, some of my earliest memories are of cowering in the furthest recesses of an understairs cupboard.
>
> But now, since the autism diagnosis, it's like having my own little rottweiler! When you're this tired, and facing so much stress, it's amazing how much it helps.>>
>
> Mack

The cystogram appointment was straightforward and very quick – we were done and dusted within half an hour. And later that day, we got a call saying the results were great so the catheter could come out as planned. Roll out the bunting!

I heard the heartening sound of Mack whistling when he was getting up next morning – something that's not happened in a long time. It's fantastic – a week and a half on from the surgery and his frame of mind still seems to be very upbeat. Unless of course he's simply masking or trying to cheer himself up – like a German doing laughing practice.

As ever, we arrived at the car park at least half an hour early and had a fair bit of time to kill before checking in for the next appointment. And then we had to kill a good deal more, as they were running behind even by 10am. That's a killer of course, a delay. But a heady cocktail of diazepam, propranolol, pacing, stimming, masking and clowning around with the other waiting gents got him by and, eventually, it was Mack's turn.

Having built himself up for an excruciating extraction, he was relieved to discover that parting with the catheter was a slithery non-event. Even better, he passed the voiding test with flying colours. Well, by something like 3ml. While that was the result *I* was expecting, my catastrophising Autie was, of course, busy worrying he'd fail and that he'd need to have the catheter put back without anaesthetic because of the propranolol. And perhaps he was right to worry – after all, none of the other guys in the waiting room were managing to pee at all. So he came home feeling rather smug. Much like a toddler who's been awarded a gold star during potty training.

Today wasn't such a good day though. Everything was going swimmingly until mid-morning when an Amazon delivery arrived. Mack had gone for a rest, and when the doorbell sounded it woke him with a start from the depths of a horrific nightmare brought on by having been on diazepam and propranolol for two days running. He leapt out of bed, confused and disorientated, and came over all dizzy as his blood pressure crashed and heart raced. A stark reminder that he not only has a long haul ahead in terms of his physical recovery from surgery, but he still needs to address the PTSD.

For now though, we're just taking one day at a time.

Back to life

The crash and burn

30 April

It's been amazing to learn all about autism and see Mack's life in a whole new light. But it's not just his *life* that has a new perspective, it's the stone wall too.

In the very first paragraph of the foreword, I described the catalyst for getting a diagnosis as being the fallout from having hit the wall, probably giving the mistaken impression that it was a sudden impact. But that's not actually how it happened. The effect was just as devastating, but the crash unfolded in protracted slow motion.

Now that we're drawing to the end of our investigations, we can see more clearly that Mack had been squaring up to that wall for probably his whole life, punching away at it – every knock taking more and more out of him – until eventually he found himself collapsed in a listless heap at its foot.

So what was it? It doesn't fit the bill of a nervous breakdown as it wasn't sudden, and it can't be explained simply in terms of anxiety or depression either.

Burnout perhaps? But according to Mental Health UK, burnout is a state of physical and emotional exhaustion caused by long-term stress in your job or when you've worked in a physically or emotionally draining role for a long time. So that's not it either, as in Mack's case it's little or nothing to do with his occupation.

There's certainly been a fire of some kind going on, but it's been a very slow burning one – and all we have left now are a few smouldering embers.

Well, it turns out there's something called *autistic* burnout. According to the National Autistic Society, "Autistic burnout is a syndrome conceptualised as resulting from chronic life stress and a mismatch of expectations and abilities without adequate supports. It is characterised by pervasive, long-term… exhaustion, loss of function, and reduced tolerance to stimulus."[27]

This sounds much more like Mack's experience – complete mental and physical fatigue to the point where he'd become barely able to function. Not surprising after a lifetime of sensory sensitivity and masking.

>   <<I had no idea what was happening to me, or why. I was just aware that every day I struggled more than the last and there were so many things I simply couldn't face any more. And it's not just the exhaustion – I've felt so *unwell* all the time. Like there's never a part of me that doesn't hurt anymore.>>
>
>   Mack

It's interesting to hear other Auties talking about this. While most of them are way younger than Mack, they still talk about the long-term effects of living in what they call permanent crisis mode and what happens when the bubble bursts and they simply don't have enough energy to carry

---

[27] National Autistic Society (2022), Understanding autistic burnout. Accessed April 2023 at:
https://www.autism.org.uk/advice-and-guidance/professional-practice/autistic-burnout

on. BBC Sounds' *1800 Seconds on Autism* talked about this during a podcast with Autie comedian Fern Brady[28].

According to Autie co-host Jamie Knight, "...there's a certain pattern for a lot of autistic people where they have a successful mask for 10 or 15 years... the burnout hits, the mask drops, and they're suddenly dealing with a level of impairment that seems to come completely out of nowhere." Nail on the head, or what? Only in Mack's case, replace 10 or 15 years with 50-odd.

During our investigations, we came across a book called *Avoiding Anxiety in Autistic Adults*[29], which looked at the subject of autistic burnout – or *crashing* as author Dr Beardon termed it. He specifically mentioned this in relation to age saying, "There are certainly some individuals for whom years of living with anxiety without any meltdown/shutdown eventually leads to a massive episode that might even be misunderstood within the context of psychiatric illness."

He suggests that while the crash is the result of decades of anxiety, it can sometimes be triggered by a lifestyle change – such as retirement, bereavement or moving home. Yep – all three apply in Mack's case. And he further noted the large numbers with health issues such as chronic fatigue or fibromyalgia – yes and yes again – saying, "The impact that being in an ongoing state of fight or flight without actually being able to do either most of the time, must surely increase the chances of there being a physiological outcome."

---

[28] BBC Sounds (2021), 1800 Seconds on Autism: Fern Brady on her recent autism diagnosis. Accessed April 2023 at:
https://www.bbc.co.uk/programmes/p097ykp6
[29] Beardon, Dr L (2021), Avoiding Anxiety in Autistic Adults: A Guide for Autistic Wellbeing. London and Boston, Sheldon Press.

He may never have met Mack, but it appears that he's met a good few of his doppelgangers.

So it looks as though anxiety may lie at the root of Mack's crash – although autistic fatigue is surely also culpable. Autistic fatigue is a term used to describe the exhaustion caused by any or many of the autistic traits we've covered – including sensory overload. We've already talked about the effort it must take to mask all the time, so this would also contribute to the fatigue and is worth looking at more closely.

Another book we found, *Autism and Masking*[30], talked about different types of masking and the adverse effects of long-term masking.

Mack jumped off the pages as being what they called an extroverted masker. This is where, rather than hiding yourself away as a result of any anxieties, you adopt a character or persona much as an actor plays a part. That character is the confident, outgoing person you probably wish you were, and that's how you portray yourself to others pretty much all the time. Presenting yourself this way not only lulls others into believing the part you're playing – it distracts you from any anxiety you may be feeling. Presumably because it's such hard work to keep it up!

The book drew parallels with undercover work. Someone who operates undercover has to learn their part inside out, remaining alert at all times to the dangers of slipping up. They need to blend in, and they can't afford to let their

---

[30] Sedgewick, Dr F; Hull, Dr L, Ellis, H (2022), Autism and Masking: How and why people do it, and the impact it can have. London, Jessica Kingsley Publishers.

concentration drop for a moment in case they fall out of character.

It also talked about method acting, where an actor assumes the persona of the character they're portraying and keeps it up not just during the shooting of a scene, but for the entire duration of the film-making. Method acting draws on aspects of yourself and your own experiences and applies them to the character you're playing. But it's been found that the performance comes at a cost – it can take a real toll on your mental health.

What's more, there was a suggestion that suppressing your own personality by pretending to be someone else can actually make you feel bad about yourself. Not great for your self-esteem or sense of self-worth.

The authors' conclusion was that long-term masking can be linked to difficulties not only with mental health but with burnout, relationships and even your sense of identity.

If you add in a good measure of the crap life throws at you from time to time anyway, and a generous splash of sensory sensitivity, it's perhaps not surprising that Mack pretty much ground to a halt.

> <<It's a double-edged sword. Masking helped me hugely throughout life, but the cost was that others believed your façade, and I found they just couldn't – or wouldn't – believe that you were struggling and needed help.
>
> For example, from the get-go I kept trying to encourage the team to bring in new business or upsell services to existing clients. They'd say things like, "I'm no good at 'marketing' – you're so much better at that." And at the same time, they'd want a raise!

> So I introduced an incentive scheme. I explained that there was only so much in the pot, but if they brought in more business, increasing the size of the pot, they'd get a share of it. It didn't make any difference though – all our new business came through my own efforts and my own contacts at an ever-increasing cost to my wellbeing.>>
>
> Mack

A while back, we watched a programme called *Paddy and Christine McGuinness: Our Family and Autism*[31]. During the filming, Christine was diagnosed as autistic and talked about her surprise when she realised just how much she masked even with her then-husband Paddy. Which of course made me question how much Mack masks with me. It's alarming to think that someone can't relax completely even in their own home.

I appreciate that if you mask all the time, it's easier to stay in character. But I can't get my head round the level of effort that must require, day in day out. While Mack admits he masks with me too, at least he doesn't do it constantly. But he does still perform for everyone else for the most part – even the kids. It's so engrained that I don't think he can switch it off, even though the kids are hugely supportive and understanding.

Maybe, just *maybe*, things will be different now.

---

[31] BBC iPlayer (2021), Paddy and Christine McGuinness: Our Family and Autism. Accessed December 2022 at:
https://www.bbc.co.uk/iplayer/episode/m00122vl/paddy-and-christine-mcguinness-our-family-and-autism

Beyond the wall

1 May

Now that we better understand the causes of Mack's crash (or "massive episode" as described by Dr Beardon), it would be helpful to know more about the road to recovery. How do we get Mack from where he is now – virtually agoraphobic – back to being able to go on long walks or a holiday again, for example?

Unfortunately, I can't find much at all on major crashes like Mack's. Even the official definition of autistic burnout describes long-term exhaustion as being from as little as '3+' months. We're a whole dimension beyond that! We need to be looking at the experiences of other people aged 55+ who have hit car-stopper walls after decades of successfully hiding their autistic anxiety without any of these wee '3+' month shutdowns.

But there's very little research out there about autism and ageing – and therefore about major, later-life crashes and recovering from them. There's a clear consensus that, while autism itself doesn't change over time, the symptoms can get worse. There are also suggestions that ageing can be much more traumatic and challenging for Auties because, compared to neurotypical people, they generally become less flexible, suffer more sensory issues and find their social skills declining faster over time. (The cancer certainly hasn't helped.)

Our experience supports the suggestion that ageing is an issue. I don't mean the silver hair and rickety knees – I guess we *can* do something about those. No, I'm thinking of psychological resilience – our ability to deal with daily stress and disturbance as we get older.

Age tends to be accompanied by a gradual decline in physical abilities and by a proliferation of health conditions. For an Autie – certainly for Mack – the decline in strength and fitness is a downer in itself. And when you add an illness like cancer to the mix, with a good dollop of uncertainty and medical anxiety, you're on the express train to depression, catastrophising all the way.

While you can live with and indeed recover from many age-related illnesses and conditions, it's clear how it would take a toll on your resilience. And this may partly explain why Mack's burnout has lasted so long with no immediate signs of recovery.

There are lots of ideas out there about how to alleviate the autism symptoms brought on by such problems – most of them already picked up throughout our journal.

I did find one gem of a blog article though, by Dr Neff, called *Autistic Burnout Recovery: How to Build a Recovery Plan*[32], which said: "If you are a high-masking autistic person or recovering from late-in-life autistic burnout, you may need more than rest and added accommodations. You may need to restructure your identity as you incorporate your neurodivergent identity."

The blog confirmed my suspicion that, given Mack's been ignoring his sensory issues, masking and over-functioning for a lifetime, his recovery is unlikely to happen overnight and… Oh. Sorry, now I'm having an epiphany…!

I've just realised I need to revisit my idea of recovery. I began this section by asking "How do we get Mack from

---

[32] Neurodivergent Insights (2022), Autistic Burnout Recovery: How to Build a Recovery Plan. Accessed May 2023 at: **https://neurodivergentinsights.com/blog/autistic-burnout-recovery**

where is now… *back* to being able to…", only to realise that this is entirely the wrong question, as it suggests he would or should be trying to get back to doing things he was managing to do before. But the whole point is that he never was. Managing it before, I mean. He was just masking. Pretending. Enduring. Over-functioning. And that's what caused the burnout in the first place. Getting back on the bus – and going to parties and restaurants and on holidays – would simply result in another crash.

So we need to reframe the question. It's not about getting *back* to doing things – which is all about keeping everyone else happy – it should be about getting to a place that makes *him* happy. Let's try "How do we get Mack from where he is now… to being able to do the things *he* wants to do?" Gosh. Now I need a lie down.

2 May

Truth be told, Mack has never enjoyed a long walk unless it's with a dog. OK, maybe we can get a dog. As for holidays, if Mack has a dog to keep him company at home, maybe I could jet off to sunny climes with Marnie from time to time…

Meantime, we should get back to focusing on a future full of whatever Mack finds restful and fulfilling. Because, while we may not need to rebuild the wall, we *do* need to rebuild Mack. How are we going to do that? Well, from all we've learned over the past few weeks and months, it seems that relaxation is going to be the key.

One of my friends found her autistic teenager smoking weed in his room one day last year and was a little taken aback. As well you might be. His answer to the obvious question, 'why?' was quite simply that it relaxed him. Or, more specifically, he said, "It's the only time I ever feel relaxed."

I guess that means he experiences life much the same way Mack does, constantly feeling that underlying anxiety.

While there seems to be general agreement among Auties that drugs are not the best way to go, we did joke after this about sending my 85-year-old mother out to buy some weed for Mack to try. She's the only person I know who knows where to get some, as she's forever complaining to the powers that be about the open dealing/smoking that goes on behind her garden wall!

However, we do believe we've found the way forward. The diagnosis was the catalyst, and the exploration we've been on ever since has helped us better understand both Mack and how we can get our lives back on track in a new, more Autie friendly world.

Strategies for Mack

3 May

Not all coping strategies work for every Autie, because every Autie is different. But here's a summary of the things that work for Mack. Sometimes at least.

Reducing sensory issues
- Be well rested before venturing out anywhere that may expose you to sensory sensitivities.
- Avoid places with overbright or fluorescent (flickering) lights.
- Keep sunglasses handy.
- Avoid crowded, noisy, and/or echoey places.
- Use active noise-reducing earplugs to muffle background sounds.
- Check the forecast and dress for the temperature and conditions.
- Keep spare jumpers and jackets in the car.
- Choose a seat in a restaurant/bar with a corner or wall behind you if possible so that noise only comes from one direction.
- Make sure there's a clear path for making a quick exit if necessary.
- Find out where the loos are – or any other quiet place – in case you need a quick rest break.
- Take a rest break or quiet time whenever you need it.
- Allow enough recovery time after your outing before scheduling another.

Keeping well
- Take quiet time to practise reading your body's signals occasionally.

- Set reminders to drink throughout the day and make sure you do actually drink.
- Eat at regular times throughout the day.
- Maintain a healthy, nutritional, balanced diet suited to your own physiological needs and accounting for any intolerances/gastrointestinal issues.
- When tired, eat something more – it's the brain telling you that you need glucose. Or possibly water.
- When your memory or ability to think is impaired, you're overtired. Eat and drink something and rest. Remember rest isn't a reward, it's a necessity.
- Schedule regular exercise.
- Do regular stretching exercises to ease off tension in the neck, shoulders and body.
- Make sure you get enough downtime, relaxation, enjoyment and sleep.
- Use a SAD syndrome light on dark winter days.
- Keep a journal – a place for venting, contemplation and keeping track.
- Give yourself permission to consign unnecessary stresses to the chuck-it bucket.

Sleeping well
- Make sure you don't eat or drink anything after 4pm that's stimulating or likely to cause heartburn.
- Don't stare at electronic screens (particularly smartphones or computers) in the run up to bedtime, as the blue light affects your melatonin levels making it harder to drift off.
- Ventilate the bedroom and keep it cool.
- Invest in a comfortable pillow that supports your head and neck and doesn't overheat you.
- Wind down before bedtime – shrug, stretch, relax, have a bath, whatever it takes.

- Empty your mind, and try some relaxation exercises or lavender if you don't fall asleep quickly.
- If your mind won't stop buzzing, write down whatever's bothering you so you can then deal with it in the morning. Keep a pen and pad (the 'park-it' pad) beside the bed.

Relaxing
- Listen to music.
- Play the piano. Or viola.
- Read, play a game or do any other enjoyable activity.
- Have a good laugh – by joking with someone, or watching or reading something funny.
- Research and plan something to look forward to.
- Do your favourite relaxation or mindfulness exercises.
- Meditate – nothing beats an empty mind and a view of the water.
- Luxuriate in a lovely warm CBD candle-lit bath to some favourite music.
- Have a small glass of red wine with dinner.
- Go for a massage occasionally.

Dealing with social events or interactions
- Carry an emergency kit with all the things you may need to avoid a meltdown, such as: earplugs, sunglasses, something to stim with, paracetamol, calm-me-down stuff, lavender stick, water and glucose, sweeties or chocolate.
- Don't forget your autism card and radar key which gives you access to public toilets.
- Dress for the occasion so you feel like you have a suit of armour.
- Schedule sufficient rest time before and after the event to prepare and recover from it.

- Allow plenty time to get there so you're not flustered and anxious about being late.
- Take a rest break if and when you're flagging, and count, breathe or stim if you start to feel anxious.
- Make sure there's a clear path for making a quick getaway if necessary.
- If it's too much, simply explain you're not feeling well and leave. Use the recuperative items from your emergency kit (water and glucose) and then rest/sleep.

Dealing with the unknown

- Research what to expect as thoroughly as possible – find out everything you can about what, where, who, how and when in advance.
- Counter any catastrophising by putting things in context/perspective – this can hugely reduce the perceived risk.
- Look for ways to turn a worry around or find something positive in it to reduce the anxiety.
- Familiarise yourself with a new environment by exploring it online first. If in doubt, call ahead.
- Depending on the situation, consider whether a desensitising approach to tackling it would help.
- If appropriate, explain to others your need to know what to expect (particularly for the likes of medical appointments).

Staving off meltdowns

- Assess a new situation to set your expectations, and then prepare for it.
- Use anything you need from your emergency kit.
- Hum a tune or listen to some calming music.
- Count slowly, breathe deeply, pace gently, adopt whatever stimming method might be handy (cornelian

stone in pocket), stretch off your neck and shoulders to ease the tension.
- Try box breathing[33]: breathe in while counting to four slowly and hold for four seconds, slowly exhale through your mouth for four seconds, repeat until you feel re-centred.
- Get away from the environment or situation that's creating the potential for meltdown.
- Call a calm person to help ground yourself.
- Monitor your heart rate and blood pressure and 'will' them down while counting, breathing, etc. But don't overdo it.

Staving off dark thoughts
- Identify probable causes and challenge negative thoughts.
- Check your water, glucose and B12 levels.
- Distract yourself with calming/relaxing/pleasant things, like playing or listening to positive music.
- Try relaxation techniques – meditation, interoception exercises.
- Use the SAD lamp, go for a walk, cuddle a puppy or person.
- Eat, sleep, cry, and/or talk to someone.

Journaling

<<Shortly after I received my autism diagnosis, I started keeping a journal. I thought it would be a good way to get my head straight, given my whole world was

---

[33] WebMD (2023), What Is Box Breathing? Accessed May 2023 at:
https://www.webmd.com/balance/what-is-box-breathing

turning upside down, and several months on I'm still finding it helpful.

It's evolving though. When I first started the journal I was feeling down, redundant, poorly, exhausted, frustrated… and I used it to write about the way I was feeling both health-wise and emotionally. Gradually, as I started to write more, it began to switch from focusing on feelings such as anger and isolation to more constructive things such as what I've done in the day and things I've got to do the following day. I'm seeing it as a bit of a progression.

Interestingly, I've found the brighter the day, the brighter my mood.

Days when I'm having problems continue to be more inward than outward looking – but the journal is a place to park ideas that are frustrating me. If I'm feeling crappy, I write it down because after a while nobody wants to hear/listen and it can be a good place to have a no-holds-barred meltdown!

However, the difficulty with a journal is I'm worried that if something happens to me, people might read it. So I'm being quite careful about what I say and I'm also using it to make sure if anyone did read it that they'd also know how much they mean to me. >>

Mack

Hmm, I'm pretty sure that vetting the content isn't the best way to get the most out of journaling. Isn't the whole point meant to be that you're free to express yourself in your own private, safe space?

I've suggested to Mack that he writes his vitriol separately and he can then consign it to the chuck-it bucket – or shred it! – after he's finished venting. That way, he gets to purge his system of the bile without having to worry about upsetting anyone. Given his listening skills, I may have to suggest this many times of course.

I'm glad he's finding journaling helpful though, and an added benefit is its use as a record. For example, this week he was looking at all the entries that mentioned migraine to figure out whether there might be a common trigger. And he'd noted days when he'd been having tingling lips which helped him identify tomato as the culprit. As if our diet wasn't limited enough!

Giving himself permission to be himself

We used to tease Halle about her dislike of having different foods on her plate touching each other – her peas or beans would need to be separated from her chips by a wall of fish fingers, for example. I had a friend like that at uni. Dugald. He not only separated his food, but ate it in a specific order too. His burger first, then the roll it had been in, then the beans, then the chips – every lunch time, day after day. He became an actuary, so the chances are high that he was an Autie too! Sorry, digressing.

I'd never noticed Mack doing the not-touching or eating-in-a-certain-order thing with his food, except for petit pois. They're always ostracised and left till last. However, since he's been 'outed' – at least among family and friends – Mack definitely seems to feel freer about indulging in this whim, so I suspect it's an inclination that he's spent his whole life stifling till now. It's great to see that instead of worrying about being odd, Mack is now embracing these strange little compulsions. After all, who cares what others think anymore?

A lot of the Autie blogs and articles I've read mention that it's important to give yourself permission to be yourself; to remove the mask and simply be who you are whenever you can. And if that means party-pooping, eating your pudding before your starter, and ranting all the way through *Politics Today*, well, it's your life, so why not?

I very much hope Mack will embrace more such 'freedoms' and not feel the same pressure to continually mask anymore. While I've not seen any change in the amount of masking he does just yet, perhaps over time...

Strategies for me

4 May

My first and main reason for writing this 'exposé' of Mack's Autie foibles was to help me figure out how best to support him. So far, I've come up with a bunch of ideas I've been trying out.

Mood monitoring

In a previous job, we used to start the day with quick, stand-up team meetings called jumpstarts, and first on the agenda would be chat; 'how is everyone today?' The point of the meetings was as much to waken and gee people up for the day as to discuss the workload. It seems like a perfectly sensible way to go about retirement life too!

While I'm already in the habit of asking Mack how he is each morning, I've started to go one step further. I've drawn up a checklist to help me to support him depending on his answer – an aide memoire that I expect will evolve over time.

If his answer is 'great', and he really does seem in good fettle, the checklist simply says:

- Don't overdo it.
- Keep drinking.
- Keep eating.
- Do something enjoyable.
- Keep taking rests.

So my job for the day is to prompt him along those lines if and when he starts to go astray!

If his reply is 'tired', his sleep monitor will tell us how well or badly he slept the night before which could explain why.

If it's not simply lack of sleep, it may be that it's his mood or that he's physically run down. Perhaps we need to give this one more thought but, for now, the checklist just says:

- Eat or drink.
- Take a powernap.
- Do you need some B12?!

For 'tense', we need to have a look at the day's schedule for a possible explanation. Regardless, this checklist may help ease his tension:

- Stretch off neck/shoulders.
- Do some physical exercise.
- Do mindfulness exercises.
- Put worries in context.
- Have a bath.
- Listen to or play music.
- Meditate.
- Have a laugh.
- Book a massage.

For 'anxious', again we need to check the schedule because the most likely explanation is going to be something we've got planned for that day. So this checklist says:

- Pass the buck – by which I mean let me do for him whatever it is that's making him anxious.
- Breathe, count, pace, stim.
- Sniff some lavender or other calming scent.
- Do you need some calm-me-down stuff?
- Review the 'tense' bullets.
- Turn worries around, looking for something positive or reassuring.
- Change your environment.

- Speak to a calm person (me, his son Stuart, my sister Marnie…).
- Rest.

For 'depressed':

- Use the SAD lamp.
- Do you need B12?
- Plan something nice.
- Go for a walk.
- Cuddle a puppy or person.
- Do a favourite activity.
- Comfort eat.
- Comfort buy – though perhaps we should have a price limit on this one!
- Review 'tense' and 'anxious' bullets.
- Have a good cry.
- Sleep.

And for 'awful':

- Consider probable causes.
- Eat, drink and sleep.
- Do you need a remedy?
- Review previous checklist bullets.
- Phone a friend or helpline.

At some stage I guess this will all become second nature and simply a routine way of keeping day-to-day life on an even keel.

Keeping in touch with friends

Mack has often said he doesn't have any friends, but that's not true. Many people have made overtures of friendship over the years but because he's met them in a professional context, he hasn't recognised these as being anything other than good working relationships. Undoubtedly, some of them consider Mack a friend and would be there for him if ever he picked up the phone. Which, to be fair, he acknowledges when I point this out.

And then there's extended family – though maybe not the cousin who told him at his mother's funeral that he'd been a horrendous child. (He *really* didn't need to hear that.)

I need to encourage him to keep in contact with them all – especially now that he's entering retirement. This is a case of the pot and kettle again though, as I'm not the best at keeping in touch myself!

I'm thinking the best approach might be to list these friends and then put automated reminders in Mack's calendar to serve as prompts. For example, "When was the last time you spoke to Calum?" or "Time to arrange coffee with Katherine." It would be a tragedy to lose touch with any of them.

The little things

I mentioned before that Mack would do anything for his family – he's pretty much always putting us and what he thinks we might like or want before himself and his own needs. So, despite the fact that we've been on this journey together and he now understands what he should and shouldn't do for the sake of his wellbeing, it's going to be hard to change this default setting.

For example, I had a hideously big birthday approaching, and he was talking about having a party. We'd barely begun to put humpty together again, *and* he was just about to begin cancer treatment – yet he was prepared to put himself through a *party*?! Luckily for him, I'd rather have a hole in the head than a party.

But it does illustrate that I'm going to have to work at least as hard as him on his wellbeing renovation. I think the key things I need to remember are:

- Continue to use and develop the morning checklists until this is second nature.
- Take any sensory concerns seriously – this is a superpower after all.
- Be very aware of environments likely to cause him sensory issues. Avoid them if at all possible and, if not, make sure we have an emergency kit to hand with his earplugs, etc.
- For back-up, keep an emergency kit in my bag or car so we're never caught without something that could help. My emergency kit currently contains earplugs, an eye mask and paracetamol, propranolol, anti-histamine, glucose, mints, photos of the kids and a tiny bottle of his happy smell.
- Even in a sensory friendly environment, make sure he can sit in a corner or with his back to a wall with a clear route to an exit.
- If he seems tired, give him a sugar boost. If it's not that, he'll be in need of water and/or a rest.
- If he's tense, anxious, depressed… use the checklists to figure out how to help.
- Remind him occasionally to do the exercises to improve his interoception – especially if he's forgetting to eat or drink, or is having problems telling whether he's hot or cold.
- Make sure he's eating and drinking at least whenever I am – bearing in mind there's more of him to fuel!
- Be aware how tired he's likely to be after social interactions of any length and make sure he gets enough rest – he's not great at resting. Nor at listening to me nagging him to rest!

- Adopt a surreptitious ear-stroking signal to let him know when he's missing end-of-conversation cues or if he's not listening enough/talking over people too much.
- Remember that listening isn't his greatest forté. If I want him to know something important, make sure he's registered it. Or write it down.
- Plan everything well and keep a schedule visible so that we can both clearly see at a glance what's happening when. Make sure 'events' are well spaced out with clear days between them for recovery. We've been using a whiteboard in our study for this.
- Join him in doing interoception and relaxation exercises – they must surely be good for me too.
- Encourage him to take time-outs or super-catnaps and facilitate that as much as possible.
- Try to arrange social 'events' at home or in another familiar environment rather than somewhere new if possible.
- When he's getting wound up, don't just tell him it's OK. Give him practical assurances that will help him to rationalise rather than catastrophise.
- Remember that he needs as much love and attention as the grandpuppies!
- Plan tummy friendly meals together and shop accordingly. Don't let the stuff of heartburn over the door.
- Research medical matters with him so that we're both on the same page, and help him with any planning and prep.
- Scope out new places or situations in advance.
- If something's wrong, and depending on what it is, try to fix it before I tell him about it.
- Look out for perseverating thoughts or behaviours that might indicate he's needing help.

- Keep steering him towards positive, rewarding and enjoyable activities and projects.
- Keep encouraging him to play the piano or viola, and also to listen to music around the house or in the car more often.
- Allow for his need to be early, and remember to account for this when setting my own expectations.
- Consider getting a puppy of our own.

Explaining it to others

6 May

Back in the foreword, I talked about finding a concise way to explain Mack's autism to friends and family. That was my second reason for embarking on this journey.

Well, those closest to us pretty much know already and have been on at least parts of this journey with us. And given he'd been knocking around this world for 63 years without ever knowing he was autistic, he probably doesn't really need to tell anyone else.

But if we *are* asked about it – or feel the need to explain his earplugs or disappearing trick – here's how we're describing it – with as much emphasis on upsides as downsides:

1. Autism simply means the brain is wired differently. For example, an Autie's ability to process what they see is 10 times *more* powerful than a neurotypical person's, although their ability to process what they hear is 10 times *less* powerful.
2. Mack experiences hypersensitivity. His brain can sometimes go into overload trying to process vast amounts of sensory information that neurotypical brains filter out automatically. Because of that, he doesn't cope well with busy or noisy environments and tries to avoid them. And sometimes he wears earplugs or sunglasses to reduce what they call sensory overload.
3. It can be very exhausting but there are huge upsides too. Auties are generally very creative and great at problem-solving because they think differently, and they're often gifted too.

Despite the fact that anxiety is a huge part of Mack's autism, this explanation doesn't touch on it.

<<I don't have a problem talking about anxiety with someone who's likely to be understanding, or who suffers from it themselves sometimes. But most people of my generation or older were brought up with old-school attitudes like 'pull yourself together' and 'a good hammering never hurt anyone'. I was endlessly on the receiving end of that philosophy and so I won't go there with judgy people like that.

The younger generation tend to be much more open-minded. They've been brought up to be more aware of mental health issues such as stress and anxiety, to be more tolerant and to understand the value of diversity. If they want to know more about how autism affects me, I'd be happy to talk more about it – but only if they ask.

My own kids never cease to amaze me in respect of their ability and willingness to accept others for what they are. I just need to be careful not to overburden them. They have their own life challenges and responsibilities with work, family and caring for others, and I couldn't be prouder of them.>>

Mack

The future

8 May

The year so far hasn't been easy, but now that we've got Mack through his cancer surgery, we're over the worst and will be taking the time over the coming weeks and months to focus on his recovery. When he's well enough, the next step will be to get help for his PTSD. All being well, a year from now he should be in a very much better place.

Having made some sense of Mack and his life – at long last! – we need to look at creating a brighter, more Autie friendly future. Learning how to manage the downsides of his autism has been a huge step forward for us both, but the real trick will be to find ways to make the most of the *upsides* and ensure Mack's retirement is a positive and enjoyable experience.

How? Well, that's a good question and it brings me back to Dr Neff's point about Mack needing to restructure his identity in light of his autism diagnosis. It's not just about managing any downsides of his autism on a day-to-day basis – that's a given. It's also about recognising that he doesn't need to adhere to neurotypical norms or expectations and that he has the right to be himself. To fulfil his own needs and wants rather than continually focusing on pleasing other people. To do what matters to *him* and makes *him* happy.

Climate activist Greta Thunberg, who was diagnosed during childhood, believes being different is a "superpower". While she admitted that autism had limited her in her earlier years – clearly recalling a time when she had no energy, no friends and didn't speak to anyone – she also said, "All of that is gone now, since I have found a meaning."[34] And I believe that's exactly where the answer lies – for Mack to find his own meaning in his post-diagnosis, post-career, post-cancer world.

> <<I'm not sure just yet what I'll do with my life now, but I know that my loves and strengths lie in music, family and helping others, and I'm sure that's where I'll 'find my happy'. I just need a little time to refocus and appreciate my new lease of life.
>
> Watch this space.>>
>
> Mack

---

[34] Greta Thunberg (2019), Instagram, Facebook, Twitter.

Epilogue

Fast forward 10 months

10 March

So how have we been getting on? Sadly, not as well as I'd hoped. The euphoria Mack felt at still being alive after surgery – and cancer-free – didn't last for very long. The realities of post-prostatectomy life hit hard and it's fair to say he felt a bit cheated that all the focus around treatment had (understandably) been on its life-saving outcome rather than its life-limiting impact.

> <<For someone in my clinical state, the risk of incontinence is supposed to be 20% ("About 20 in 100 men have this issue after 6 years") and the risk of erectile dysfunction is supposed to be 50% ("About 50 in 100 men have this issue after 6 years")[35]. But the devil is in the small print; i.e. the definitions of incontinence and erectile dysfunction. No one actually said that, even for the lucky ones, life would never be the same again. And that's been indescribably hard to deal with.
>
> I know, I need to get it in perspective. Am I glad to be alive?... I think so. Yes. Most days...>>
>
> Mack

---

[35] University of Cambridge (2022), Predict Prostate. Accessed November 2022 at:
https://prostate.predict.cam/tool

It's been hard to see Mack in such a dark place for so long. But they did say it would be a long road to recovery. We're not yet one year on never mind *six* years, and I just need to keep reminding him of that and support him as best I can through the black times.

Thankfully, it's not *all* been doom and gloom. There have been three sunny rays cutting through the darkness that are making – and will increasingly make – a huge difference. First, Tamara the cockapoo. Second, brand new grandson Elliot. And third, counsellor Suneeta.

To Tamara first of all.

Last summer, Marnie, Grady and I met a guy with a lovely wee dog called Spike. We couldn't make out what kind of dog Spike was, so of course just had to ask. "He's a cockapoo!" his owner was delighted to tell us. "I could only have a poodle cross really because my wife is allergic to everything from hamsters to horses, but she's fine with Spike." *Really*?! I thought. Because I'm allergic to everything too. When I'd half-heartedly said before that maybe we could get a puppy, for me that would have meant reconciling myself to a life of sneezing, wheezing and speaking with a deep husky voice. So this was a revelation.

After a bit of research, Mack and I decided a cavapoo was probably the right answer for us, so we arranged to visit a nearby breeder and snuffle some puppies. Just to be sure. They were gorgeous, but tiny – and because their dad was a toy poodle, they would always be quite tiny. Cute, but Mack didn't really want to walk a handbag. And while we were humming and hawing, we met Tamara the cockapoo.

We'd ruled out a cockapoo as an option because being descended from a cocker spaniel would have meant it was as mad as Haggis. And while we love Haggis to bits, we figured he was a bit much for us oldies to handle full-time. "Oh, but Tam's a miniature cockapoo," the breeder told us, "You'd be fine with her." …Tam? *Tam*?! Say no more, it was a sign. Mack missed his dad so much, there was absolutely no doubt that Tam would be coming home with us! It was *meant* to be.

In truth, Mack wasn't well enough to take on a puppy, but I promised to do all the hard work of house training, walkies and poo-pick-upping while he recovered, in the hope that he would reap all the therapy benefits of puppy cuddles.

I won't pretend it's been plain sailing. Sometimes Mack has been so down that he's had no bandwidth for even a well-behaved wee bundle of cheek, and her presence has made him feel "trapped". Other times, he's credited her with being a life-saver because there's nothing quite like being loved by a cockapoo when you just want to cry your eyes out.

What's more, she's a hoot. For Christmas, she was given some of those 'talking dog' buttons that are meant to help dogs tell you want they want. You record a key word onto each button – 'Hungry', 'Go pee' and 'Walkies' for example – and once she's learned the words, she's supposed to press the appropriate button rather than just badger, bounce and bark at you.

She's still learning of course, but getting there. The day before yesterday, she tried to tell us she wanted to go outside firstly by knocking over my wellies and then tossing Mack's shoes around the room. When that failed to get our attention – we were in the middle of an important conversation – she barked at me and then went back to pointedly toying with my wellies. A few minutes later we heard Mack's voice clearly shouting 'Out!' from the back door, and then she presented herself in front of us to make sure we'd heard.

When we still didn't respond, she whacked the 'Shonagh!' button. We couldn't help but laugh, but we were still busy. Sadly, Tam has no patience, so next it was: 'Out!', 'Go poo!' 'Love you!' followed by a moment's silence – that was a new button and clearly a surprise to her – then: 'Love you! Love you! Love you!'... as she chucked the new button around the room in delight! You can't not chuckle at precociousness like that.

As I was saying, therapy for Mack was the motivation behind getting a puppy, but it's a decision that's turning out to be hugely beneficial for *me*. It's hard supporting someone who's struggling as much as Mack without sinking along with them, but having to look after a daft and cheeky wee mutt who makes you smile and obliges you to get fresh air and daily exercise is a terrific antidote. I wouldn't be without her now!

Typically, our puppy parenting plan hit the rocks one day when I woke up feeling terrible. I had a sharp pain in my abdomen which Mack decided was appendicitis, and he nagged me for hours till I eventually agreed to phone the doctor. He was right of course.

Three days later, I was discharged from hospital after having had an appendectomy – not to mention a hysteroscopy, oophorectomy, polypectomy, D&C and endometrial biopsy following the discovery of "a large mass" in my womb and cervix! So, no dog walking or poo-pick-upping for me for a while.

> <<The thought of Shonagh being ill was hard enough to deal with, but suddenly finding myself responsible for a hyperactive little cockapoo – well, I really wasn't ready for that.

The worst thing about those three days when Shonagh was in hospital was not being there for her. But she was very dismissive of that: someone had to look after Tam; it was only an appendectomy after all (or so we thought at that point); and she'd rather I focused on my own recovery than set myself back by making unnecessary hospital trips, etc, etc.

But stepping up to look after Tam was also harder than I'd imagined. No matter how badly I'd slept, I had to be up by 8am to let her outside. Then there was all the bending up and down to reach her (why, oh why did we choose such a small dog?!). And despite her size, she still felt pretty heavy to my aching abdomen.

I'll be forever grateful to Marnie and Grady who kindly took care of the dog walking while Shonagh recovered. Not only was I still fighting agoraphobia, but I've also developed 'range anxiety' as a result of the surgery. When I have to go, I have to go *now* (well, within a few minutes), so I can't be any significant distance away from a loo yet.>>

Mack

You can probably imagine how I felt when I first heard the words "we've found a large mass…"

Two thoughts sprang to mind; first, 'Oh my God, I've got late-stage cervical cancer' and, second, 'There's no way Mack can handle this on top of what he's already dealing with!' Both prospects were a little terrifying. However, the problem of how best to hide it from Mack was probably a great distraction from fretting about the implications of such a diagnosis. And luckily I had Marnie's wise counsel to keep my head in place.

Cleverly, I thought, we avoided mentioning any possibility of cancer to Mack, telling him only that a CT scan and ultrasound had shown up a cyst, polyp and fibroids. All lovely non-cancerous stuff. He took it calmly and I thought I'd got away with it. But, once back home, one of the first questions he asked was when I'd get my biopsy results. Yep, guess who'd been researching again!

(Thankfully, my results came back clear.)

14 March

The second ray of light in this last year or so has come in the form of brand new tiny human Elliot, Halle and Connor's first child. Mack's grandson.

Mack was delighted (but not overly surprised as he's been waiting a long time for this!) when Halle first told us they were having a baby. Delighted for *them* obviously, but it was also great for Mack to have something so positive to focus on. Something to look forward to. And look forward to it he did.

But timing has never been Mack's strong point, and he happened to be in the throes of PTSD therapy – yes, finally! – when Elliot arrived three weeks ago. This meant that Mack wasn't in the best of fettles for making the journey to meet the wee one, though obviously he was determined to do it regardless.

Up to this point, Mack had only ever used diazepam to help him attend a dental or medical appointment. However, his anxiety and agoraphobia are crippling at the moment and it was the only way he could make it through to Glasgow. It was worth it though, and hopefully our second and subsequent visits will be a bit easier.

18 March

I mentioned there have been three sunny rays cutting through Mack's dark clouds; the third is Suneeta.

Back in September/October, Mack had been browsing LinkedIn when he happened to notice a post from Macmillan Cancer Support aimed at people who have or have had cancer and were struggling psychologically. Well, if ever he needed psychological support, it was now! So he booked an 'emotional wellbeing assessment call' designed to help them understand the issues Mack was facing. And from there he was offered six free counselling sessions to help him come to terms with the after-effects of his surgery.

And hats off to Macmillan, they managed to find him a counsellor who also has significant experience of working with Auties.

> <<I so wasn't expecting that. To be able to speak to someone who not only understands the emotional toll cancer takes on you, but the autistic mind too? That's huge, and it took a lot of the trepidation out of that first session for me. It wasn't long before we'd established a connection and I felt at ease with Suneeta.
>
> I was lucky to get onto the programme in the first place – it proved so popular that Macmillan had to withdraw it because of funding constraints – but I feel particularly lucky to have been matched to Suneeta. Those first sessions organised by Macmillan were, for me, the perfect introduction to the perfect lifeline, as I believe Suneeta can help me with

so many aspects of my life that have led me to the dark place I've been floundering around in for so long.>>

Mack

During their initial session, back in early November, Suneeta very quickly realised that Mack's cancer was merely the tip of his iceberg. It was clear to her that many other issues lurked under the surface; such as autism, PTSD, agoraphobia, general anxiety disorder, bereavement... Not exactly a quick fix.

Those first six sessions helped raise Mack from a jet black place to somewhere dawn grey. A great start. But crucially, having established a relationship of trust with Suneeta, Mack has continued to work with her on his other challenges. I'm immensely hopeful that she'll be able to help him through the burnout and out the other side.

Along the way, she's been giving him exercises to help reframe his mindset, but also some great tips. For example, remember I mentioned that his hands would become freezing cold when he found himself approaching fight or flight, all the blood having rushed to his core in favour of heart-pumping? Suneeta suggested he try handwarmers. This draws the blood back, gradually reducing the impending panic attack. I have to say it sounded a little dubious to me at first, but he's found it really works! In fact, this is probably the most effective trick he's learned since discovering ear plugs.

24 March

When we first realised that Mack suffered from PTSD, he understandably felt he had way too much on his plate to be able to deal with it, so he 'parked' it for later. His intention had been to go back to Nicol when he felt ready. However, as his anxiety, depression and trauma are all inextricably linked, the subject of PTSD inevitably cropped up during his sessions with Suneeta. It seemed only natural then that they would work on it together. That process has only recently begun.

Expecting that this would mean things would get worse before they got better, I did a little more homework to build on my understanding of the condition. I found a lot of great sources, but the PTSD UK website particularly caught my attention because their strapline, 'Tomorrow can be a new day' resonated with me. I *so* hope this will be the case.

The website explains that, "During trauma, your brain thinks, 'processing and understanding what is going on right now is not important! Getting your legs ready to run, your heart rate up, and your arms ready to fight this danger is what's important right now, I'll get back to the processing later.' Until the danger passes, the mind does not produce a memory for this traumatic event in the normal way."

"The facts of what happened, the emotions associated with the trauma and the sensations touch, taste, sound, vision, movement, and smell can be presented by the mind in the form of flashbacks – as if they are happening right now."[36]

Right now?! I found this shocking, but also enlightening. It explains what Mack meant when he mentioned a couple of weeks ago, weirdly I thought, that Suneeta was trying to help him move from the present to the past tense.

There was worse to come though; the website went on to explain that when someone has been subjected to repeated

---

[36] PTSD UK (2024), Causes of Post Traumatic Stress Disorder. Accessed March 2024 at:
https://www.ptsduk.org/what-is-ptsd/causes-of-ptsd/

or sustained traumas or has experienced a number of different traumas, they're likely to have *complex* PTSD. Well, he never did do things by halves.

Mack had, for the most part, managed to keep a lid on the box for five decades, despite the intermittent flashbacks and nightmares which have increased in frequency since he hit the wall.

But with Suneeta's help, he has identified five particular sources of trauma from his childhood which took place before the age of 13 or 14. His abusers included both adults and older fellow pupils. While only two of the traumas were repeated, one of those was a good deal more serious and soul-destroying than the other and went on weekly for many months.

What's different in today's social environment is that these things are starting to be talked about more openly. Fellow victims have been speaking out publicly about abuse they suffered in schools, children's homes or religious institutions, either in an attempt to bring perpetrators to justice or as part of a healing process.

In July 2022, broadcaster Nicky Campbell revealed that he had witnessed and experienced sexual and violent physical abuse at his school which had had a profound effect on his life and haunted him still. And this month (March 2024), Princess Diana's brother Earl Charles Spencer released a memoir recounting the traumas of his own childhood.

Usually, news reports about things like this are about complete strangers. But when it's someone you know – albeit not personally – it seems different somehow. Closer? More real? More relatable maybe. Stories about the experiences of public figures certainly get a lot more coverage, and I think this encourages more people who have long suffered silently to speak up or seek counselling. It helps dissipate the shame and points the blame where it rightly belongs – on the perpetrators rather than the victims.

During the current long-running Scottish Child Abuse Inquiry, Nicky Campbell talked about a culture of anticipated violence and normalised sexual assault at his school – and of complicity, with teachers ignoring signs of abuse. He also talked about the heavy toll that going public about the abuse had taken on him, disrupting his sleep and causing him to seek therapy. But he also said, "This is the best decision I ever made."[37] Presumably because it's helped him lay to rest the ghost(s) that had been haunting him.

A few nights ago, I watched Earl Spencer's interview with Laura Kuenssberg on BBC iPlayer. In it, he describes the violence and sexual abuse he experienced as a child and revealed that he'd needed treatment for trauma after writing the book. The programme made for harrowing viewing.

When asked about the effect on him of finally putting pen to paper, he said, "It took me into very dark places inside of me. I had endless nightmares. I started having migraines again which I hadn't had since I was at that school. It was very bad. And then… by the end of it I was so exhausted."

"I got to a place where everything seemed rather pointless. Not suicidal, but everything seemed absolutely pointless because I think confronting – I don't think it's an

---

[37] The Guardian (2023), Nicky Campbell 'haunted' by abuse at Edinburgh Academy, inquiry hears. Accessed March 2024 at: **https://www.theguardian.com/society/2023/aug/22/nicky-campbell-scottish-child-abuse-inquiry-edinburgh-academy**

overstatement to say – confronting *evil*... well, it's cataclysmic. Or it can be."[38]

And of the system that allowed this to happen, he said, "You're going to come out very damaged, and I know I did... To survive that, a small but important part of me had to die."

It was sobering to hear him talk. Not surprising – there were echoes of Mack throughout – but I found myself sitting watching an empty screen in silence for a while afterwards.

The upside is that, having 'confronted the evil' in the way he has, Earl Spencer has finally been able to move on with his life. And, for Mack, that's exactly what I'm hoping for.

10 April

Today marked another milestone in Mack's cancer recovery; his review consultation a year on from the surgery. It's fair to say that the post-prostatectomy depression he's been struggling with is still weighing heavily on him, and I'd been hoping that this consultation would help give him a little perspective and encouragement. Has it? Hmm... on balance, probably not really.

Yes, they told him he was doing well compared to so many others. They reminded him that 'recovery' takes a long time and that it would be another year or two before he would really know his functional outcome. They even mentioned there was more they might be able to do surgically to help if, in the next year or two, there there's been no further

---

[38] BBC iPlayer (2024), Earl Spencer talks to Laura Kuenssberg. Accessed March 2024 at:
https://www.bbc.co.uk/iplayer/episode/m001xx35/earl-spencer-talks-to-laura-kuenssberg

improvement. Whoopee, more surgery. Not sure I can see that happening.

Mack listened – or at least heard – enough to be able to recount all this to me afterwards (Tam and I were waiting for him in the car park). But I'm not sure he's processed it because it hasn't exactly put a skip in his step.

> <<There's a distinct lack of support provided by the NHS in psychosexual matters after cancer surgery or treatments, which is hugely disappointing. It's left me feeling… abandoned and discarded, inadequate, incomplete, desolate… and, well, pointless really. A year on and I still find it hard to believe there's no mental health follow-up or support after you've undergone life-changing surgery.
>
> However, I've taken some comfort from the focus on this by the forthcoming International Oncology and Supportive Care Congress in Dubai which I hope will provide lessons for the UK. For an Autie especially, such support could be invaluable.>>
>
> Mack

6 May

Suneeta has been drawing on the rewind technique[39] for Mack's PTSD therapy. This is something that was first

---

[39] International Association for Rewind Trauma Therapy (2024), Rewind Therapy. Accessed May 2024 at:
https://www.iartt.com/the-rewind

introduced back in 1991 by Dr David Muss who carried out Suneeta's training.

According to PTSD UK, the rewind technique is a way of reviewing and revisiting traumatic events in a controlled and dissociative way; exposing yourself to memories without connecting to the emotional and mental impact they create[40]. Mack's autism makes this trickier than might otherwise be the case because it involves imagination and going to your 'safe space' which, as we now know, Mack can't do very well. But where there's a will there's a way!

To begin with, Suneeta worked with Mack on coping strategies so that she could be sure he would have the tools he'd need to get through the therapy – that was where the discussion about the hand warmers had come from for example, as regulating temperature is important. It was also important to establish 'grounding techniques' and desensitise 'output symptoms'. So together they talked about triggers and worked out strategies to deal with the issues.

Once she was sure that Mack would be able to cope with discussing what had happened, Suneeta decided they should focus on the two worst sources of trauma that Mack had identified. Her counselling has largely drawn on the approaches outlined in a work called *Counselling Skills for Working with Trauma: Healing From Child Sexual Abuse, Sexual Violence and Domestic Abuse*.[41]

---

[40] PTSD UK (2024), How Rewind Therapy can help people with PTSD. Accessed May 2024 at:
https://www.ptsduk.org/how-rewind-therapy-can-help-people-with-ptsd/
[41] Sanderson, C (2013), Counselling Skills for Working with Trauma: Healing From Child Sexual Abuse, Sexual Violence and Domestic Abuse. London, Jessica Kingsley Publishers.

With Suneeta's help, he's been working on feelings of helplessness, anger, guilt, revulsion and weakness, trying to replace them with something else. So now, whenever these feelings arise during a flashback or bad dream, Mack has to repeat a kind of mantra to himself to overwrite them; 'it's in the past', 'it's not happening now', 'the worst is over', 'everything will be fine', etc. Self-forgiveness is key, he tells me. (Even though – from my outsider's point of view – he doesn't have anything he needs to forgive himself for!)

Clearly, it's not easy. Mack has been fragile throughout the process and there have been some very dark days – some that have left me anxious about leaving him alone even for the time it takes to jog Tam around the block! The emotional toll of raking over it all leaves him shredded and chronically exhausted. But he did say the other day that it must be making a difference because he hasn't had a nightmare for a little while now. Hmm, let's not count our chickens just yet.

24 May

Exhaustion, or autistic fatigue, is something we've touched on a few times during this journal – usually in the context of discussing an autistic trait. We know that masking for example is exhausting. As are over-functioning and coping with sensory assault. Simply living your everyday life as an autistic person in a neurotypical world is exhausting, but when you've reached total burnout and then add illness on top of that...

Virtually every day Mack has been saying, "I just don't know what's wrong with me", as he gives me a catalogue of the day's pains and feelings of unwellness. Well, we *do* know really; we've uncovered it all in the above goodness-knows-how-many pages. He's just perseverating over it. Or is it ruminating? Anyway, it leads to more and more researching as he tries to find further explanations and potential remedies. I'm not sure that there are any more out there, but he does find comfort in reading other Auties' experiences, as they make him feel much less alone in his torment.

One had him in tears the other day; a blog on autistic fatigue and exhaustion by Undercover Autie[42]. This is how she describes her experience of it:

"I was exhausted. As someone who naturally tries to battle through an obstacle without giving it a second thought, I simply hadn't noticed. In part, I am bad at discerning my own feelings and sensations. But soldiering on is also how I coped with life… I don't tend to realise I've pushed myself too far until I collapse.

"I wake up and feel unrested. Getting my brain out of 'sleep' mode and into any kind of action feels like dredging the bottom of a lake. It's heavy and slow and muddy... I am painfully tired, physically and metaphorically, and if I don't distract myself while I go about my day, I will probably just lie down on the floor and stop moving… I, unhelpfully, start to berate myself for not doing more. Am I being lazy? Am I not trying hard enough? Deep down, I know this isn't true. I'm trying my absolute hardest, all the time."

And then at bedtime, "I'm now a weird mix of wired and tired… But I lie awake. I toss and turn for an hour, my body aching but unable to shut off."

It's not just the description of the fatigue that resonates with Mack, but the drive to continue regardless. And he also has

---

[42] Undercover Autie (2018), Autistic Fatigue and Exhaustion. Accessed May 2024 at:
https://www.undercoverautie.com/blog/2018/2/1/autistic-fatigue-and-exhaustion

trouble getting to, and staying, asleep – a double whammy given disrupted sleep can lead to increased stress!

It's interesting that other Auties experience sleep problems too. Fellow traveller Sabrina mentioned that her husband has terrible sleep and that her elder youngster is even worse – often too tired to go to bed.

We came across several 'scholarly articles' citing links between interoception and circadian rhythms/sleep cycles. Apparently interoception affects sleep, and sleep deprivation has profound effects on interoception[43]. So, sadly, Mack's interoceptive issues aren't just limited to thirst, temperature, hunger, tiredness and some emotions after all. His inability to sleep is a biggie just now.

> <<Sleep presents me with a number of problems – aches, pains and gastro issues aside.
>
> If the day has been frustrating, my brain unpacks all the things I could have said or done better, or with more impact, and stokes emotions such as anger and frustration. On the worst occasions, I can't sleep at all until an issue is dealt with. So I often find myself getting up to do a piece of work so that I can then get some rest.
>
> When I finally get over, I sleep in snatches or batches of one or two hours before I wake and feel I have to get up. Which means I then need to go through the whole routine of

---

[43] ScienceDirect (2020), Interoception relates to sleep and sleep disorders. Accessed May 2024 at:
https://www.sciencedirect.com/science/article/pii/S235215461 9301263

getting back to sleep. If and when I fall asleep straightaway, I'm fully alert again an hour and a half later.

When the room is cold, it takes me an age to get warm – I often spend two or three hours tossing and turning before sleep comes. When it's too hot, sleep is difficult as my temperature regulation doesn't work effectively. I need the covers in the same position regardless, which can then result in overheating.

Sleep analysers tell me I sleep mostly very lightly, with an average of five interruptions a night. When I'm ruminating, my heart rate can be as high as it is during the day. And a racing heart, often from things that really annoyed or worried me – like recovering from medical issues or before the dentist – can happen a few times a year.

I very seldom dream as I'm usually so tired from the day's over-thinking that there's little bandwidth left for that. Once my cancer treatment was over and healing was underway, I did have dreams for a while. Not good ones, unfortunately, but bad ones that seemed to focus on the earlier life incidents which resulted in my PTSD. It was like reliving the events in detail – seeing the faces, smelling the odours, feeling the aggression and sensations – but oddly not reliving the pain. Thankfully, likely due to counselling and refiling my memories, these dreams seem to have dried up as I haven't had one for a while now.>>

Mack

26 May

Investigating the issue of a racing heart during the night led us to an interesting article entitled *Did You Know It's Possible to Have a Panic Attack In Your Sleep?*[44]

"It's the middle of the night, you're fast asleep and suddenly – you're jolted awake. Your heart is racing, you're shaking and sweating, and it feels as though the walls are closing in around you and you can barely breathe. What the hell? You may have just experienced a specific type of panic attack, similar to a night terror, known as a nocturnal panic attack." Who knew.

Sounds like a nightmare to me, but apparently it's not. When you wake up from a nightmare, you can remember what was scaring you. But with a nocturnal panic attack, you have no memory of what caused the panic.

While it can happen to anyone, it's most common with people who have sleep disorders, who have general anxiety and panic disorder, or who suffer from PTSD-related nightmares. So, I now have my fingers tightly crossed that these incidents will stop once Mack is through the other side of his PTSD therapy. Imagine, some day soon we could both get a good night's sleep!

---

[44] Shape (2021), Did You Know It's Possible to Have a Panic Attack In Your Sleep? Accessed May 2024 at:
https://www.shape.com/lifestyle/mind-and-body/nocturnal-panic-attacks

I began this epilogue by expressing disappointment that Mack hasn't made as good a recovery as I'd hoped over the last year; that he's still in a pretty dark place and suffering from multiple aches, pains and general unwellness.

Well, today I'm feeling much more upbeat! Last night, Mack came across another article, from that same source, called *Why You Physically Feel Like Shit After Therapy*.[45] It explains that working through mental and emotional trauma can absolutely take a real physical toll.

Because trauma therapy involves facing some deep emotional issues, "…you might feel pretty beat up post-therapy. This is a very real phenomenon that you may have experienced without even noticing. Was your last migraine on the same day as your last psychotherapy visit? Did you see your therapist and feel completely depleted for the rest of the day? You're not alone. Experts from all areas of the mental health field verified that post-therapy fatigue, aches, and even physical symptoms of illness are not just real, but extremely common."

The article got a bit scientific, leaving my head spinning with mentions of cortisol, catecholamines, neurotransmitters, epinephrine, norepinephrine… However, the gist of it was that psychotherapy affects brain chemistry and this, in turn, is expressed through physical symptoms.

The most common include:

---

[45] Shape (2020), Why You Physically Feel Like Shit After Therapy, Explained by Mental Health Pros. Accessed May 2024 at:
https://www.shape.com/lifestyle/mind-and-body/physical-effects-trauma-therapy

- Gastrointestinal and gut issues.
- Headaches or migraines.
- Severe fatigue.
- Muscle aches and weakness, backaches, body aches.
- Flu-like symptoms, general malaise.
- Irritability.
- Anxiety and panic attacks.
- Mood problems.
- Sleep-related problems.
- Lack of motivation.
- Feelings of depression.

Ha! I couldn't have expressed Mack's complaints better or more comprehensively myself. Though, to be fair, he'd been experiencing a good many of those *before* therapy too. But now, when he says to me each morning, "I don't know what's wrong with me", I can just save my breath and hand him this explanation. With a smile, because I'm certain that he'll feel *so* much better when it's all behind him!

29 May

Mack is now on the third and final stage of his PTSD therapy, so it shouldn't be much longer before he begins to feel a little better, and then he'll be able to turn his attention to tackling the anxiety and agoraphobia.

Anxiety is a biggie, obviously, and it's been pretty crippling in the last couple of years. Since our initial investigations into the types of anxiety Auties are prone to, we've come across a new term – high-functioning anxiety. It's not recognised as a separate condition; it's more like a subset of general anxiety disorder. The Mayo Clinic describes it as, "when a person has anxiety symptoms, but rather than retreating from situations or interactions, they work hard to face their fears and are skilled at covering up symptoms."[46]

People with this type of anxiety disorder often excel in their professional lives and appear to be in control. They make an effort to be socially outgoing and even have strong personal relationships. But it's just a mask really. Underneath, they struggle with persistent feelings of stress, self-doubt, fears of not measuring up and of losing control – and "a sense of impending doom". They constantly strive for perfection and to please others. This doesn't just take a huge toll on their mental health, but the chronic stress involved in over-functioning tends to result in physical health problems too. "This intense push can lead to burnout because of their constant drive to overachieve and their fear of failure."

Remind you of anyone? Yep, Suneeta's got her work cut out for her, hasn't she?!

We're not expecting a miracle 'cure' for any of it. But once he's laid to rest the demons of the past, I hope Mack will have more strength to deal with the challenges that remain ahead of him. And that once he's ready to get out and about again, we'll manage his autism better. Much better. After all, we know all the tricks of the trade now, don't we?

'Out and about' is a relative term of course – we won't be doing wild parties or fly-drive city breaks any time soon. Or ever again actually. What was it I was saying before? It won't be about getting back to doing all the things Mack used to do – which was all about keeping everyone else

---

[46] Mayo Clinic (2023), Behind the mask: Managing high-functioning anxiety. Accessed May 2024 at:
https://www.mayoclinichealthsystem.org/hometown-health/speaking-of-health/managing-high-functioning-anxiety

happy – it will be about living life on his own, unashamedly autistic terms and doing all the things *he* wants to do. Hopefully that will include walking the dog. Tam would be delighted – she's such a daddy's girl.

On that note, I think we should give Tam the last word; it's the least she deserves after we ignored her woofs for attention this afternoon. We were both busy upstairs and figured she should be happy as she'd not long come back from a walk, and she'd had a lovely Lily's Kitchen cottage pie for lunch. Must be the TV she's barking at, right? Nope, turns out she needed to 'Go poo!' So, Tam's last word was actually a last turd. Right in the middle of the kitchen floor! Wee soul.

The end.

Acknowledgements

Our heartfelt thanks go to:

The Edinburgh Special Care Dentistry team. The dental counselling sessions they offered enabled Mack not only to face dental work again – with his dentist's help – but to apply the same desensitising techniques to other challenging situations. Without their help, going through cancer treatment would have been impossible for Mack.

The team and psychiatric nurse at Barclay Medical Practice in Edinburgh. At a time when pressure on GP and NHS services has never been greater, their responsiveness, sensitivity, courtesy and care has been amazing and is enormously appreciated.

The team at Number 6. The diagnosis they provided for Mack's medical file was a tremendous help to him during his cancer treatment. But, even more importantly, the late diagnosis group sessions were invaluable in helping Mack understand himself and begin to manage the downsides of his autism. Thanks also for providing detailed commentary on our text.

The Samaritans. There have been a few occasions over the last 20+ years when Mack has hit rock bottom, and their listening ear has helped him through it. Thanks to them, he's still with us.

Macmillan Cancer Support. By arranging counselling sessions for Mack to help him deal with the after-effects of his cancer surgery, they threw him a lifeline in the form of the counsellor they matched him with.

Oceanic Counselling. Mack had considered counselling before, but couldn't find anyone he could relate to or trust.

Macmillan had matched him perfectly to a counsellor with experience of working with Auties. Following the sessions provided by Macmillan, she has continued to support Mack and is helping him to slowly rebuild his life.

Prostate Cancer UK. The comprehensive information provided by this charity was instrumental in helping Mack to reach the right – for him – treatment decision. And the support provided by their specialist nurses and helpline on the occasions he called to discuss any concerns was extremely helpful.

The autistic community. Many Auties have shared their own experiences online through forums, social media and blogs, providing us with a wealth of information that hasn't yet been well researched and reported by the professionals. Having Mack's own experiences validated by those of other Auties has been immensely reassuring for him and has made him feel much less alone.

Our friends. The support of *all* our friends since Mack's diagnoses has helped hugely. Particular thanks go to: Brodie for sharing his own cancer experience with Mack, for putting Mack in touch with Chalky and for his moral support throughout; Sabrina, whose husband and elder child are both autistic and have ADHD, for sharing her thoughts and experiences with us and for her insightful commentary; and Marina, foster mother to an autistic son, also for sharing her thoughts, insights and tips!

Our family. The unwavering support of both Mack's family and my own has made these tough few years so very much easier than they might have been. Nothing beats the cushion of unconditional love and acceptance when you're feeling a little battered and bruised. As Mack says, "You're the light at the end of this tunnel."